FOOD

A Handbook of Terminology, Purchasing & Preparation

Twelfth Edition

Production Editing: Bass Communications
Design and Layout: Yondee Designs, LLC

ISBN-10: 0846100061
ISBN-13: 978-0-8461-0006-5

Printed in the United States of America

FOOD

A Handbook of Terminology, Purchasing & Preparation

Twelfth Edition

Community of Nutrition, Health, & Food Management
American Association of Family & Consumer Sciences

AMERICAN ASSOCIATION OF FAMILY & CONSUMER SCIENCES

Alexandria, Virginia
www.aafcs.org

Preface to the Twelfth Edition

The previous editions produced by volunteers of the Community of Nutrition, Health, & Food Management (NHFM) of the American Association of Family & Consumer Sciences (AAFCS) served as foundations for this revision. Many pages and much of the information remain intact, and thus we are indebted to previous authors and contributors (e.g., Dr. Carolyn Bednar, Dr. Janice Harte, Dr. Nancy Lewis, Dr. Diane McComber, and Dr. Rachel Schemmel).

Reorganizing, simplifying, and providing updated information was the focus of this project. Although digital access to materials is available via the internet, the original purpose of this handbook remains the same after 67 years: to provide valid information for the cook in a convenient format. Any comments and feedback are welcomed. Please contact AAFCS at staff@aafcs.org. For links to additional sources of information, please visit the AAFCS website at www.aafcs.org/Resources/Foodbook.asp (these were included in previous editions).

LEAD EDITOR

Anna Sumabat Turner, M.Ed., CFCS–HNFS
Leader, AAFCS Community of Nutrition, Health, & Food Management
Former Instructor, Food and Nutrition, Bob Jones University

CHAPTER EDITORS

Chapter 1: General Food Information
Carolyn Bednar, Ph.D., R.D.
Professor Emeritus, Texas Woman's University

Chapter 2: Glossary
Joanne M. Pearson, Ph.D., R.D.
Associate Professor Emerita of Health Sciences
James Madison University

Chapter 3: Milk and Milk Products
Kay M. Wilder, Ed.D., CFCS
Chairman, Department of Family & Consumer Sciences
Point Loma Nazarene University

Chapter 4: Meat
Kay M. Wilder, Ed.D., CFCS
Chairman, Department of Family & Consumer Sciences
Point Loma Nazarene University

Chapter 5: Fish and Shellfish
Claudia Sealey-Potts, Ph.D., R.D., LD
Assistant Professor
University of North Florida

Chapter 6: Poultry and Eggs
Janelle M. Walter, Ph.D., R.D., CFCS
Professor, Department of Family & Consumer Sciences
Baylor University

Chapter 7: Fruits
Lorna Hix Williams
Former South Carolina DHEC, Nutritionist III,
WIC Mother and Baby Supervisor

Chapter 8: Vegetables
Lorna Hix Williams
Former South Carolina DHEC, Nutritionist III,
WIC Mother and Baby Supervisor

Chapter 9: Grain Products
Carolyn Bednar, Ph.D., R.D.
Professor Emeritus, Texas Woman's University

Chapter 10: Sweetening Agents, Fats and Oils, Leavening Agents
Claudia Sealey-Potts, Ph.D., R.D., LD
Assistant Professor
University of North Florida

Chapter 11: Miscellaneous Foods
Joanne M. Pearson, Ph.D., R.D.
Associate Professor Emerita of Health Sciences
James Madison University

Chapter 12: Buying Guides
Sharyl Lynn Lokken Heavin, CFCS
Former Food and Nutrition Instructor, Saddleback College
Market Research, Equipment, & Test Kitchen Consultant

Chapter 13: Food Preservation
Sharyl Lynn Lokken Heavin, CFCS
Former Food and Nutrition Instructor, Saddleback College
Market Research, Equipment, & Test Kitchen Consultant

Sources of Information (online at www.aafcs.org)
Dorothy West, Ph.D.
Former Assistant Professor, Department of Family and Child Ecology
Michigan State University
Nutrition Educator

AAFCS Community of NHFM Contributors
Food Safety
Geri Banko, M.S., Nutrition
Family Consumer Sciences teacher

Microwave Information
Caryl Lokken Gonzales, M.A.
Family Consumer Sciences Teacher and Adult Educator

Table of Contents

CHAPTER 1: General Food Information

CONSTRUCTION OF RECIPES

The writing of recipes carries with it a double responsibility. First, each recipe must be accurate and complete in essentials and written simply and clearly so that it cannot be misunderstood. At the same time, it is important to present the recipe in a way that appeals to users while keeping within space limits.

A recipe is made up of two major parts — the list of ingredients and the method of preparation. Readily available ingredients, level measurements, and a simple procedure are ideal components of a recipe and should be used whenever possible. However, when the quality of a dish depends upon special ingredients or an unusual procedure, the recipe also should include this information.

The following are some well-established rules for writing or editing recipes. Guidelines for metric usage also are presented. Since the metric system is used globally, this will facilitate conversion of recipe units for diverse groups.

TABLE 1.1
TABLE OF EQUIVALENTS

ABBREVIATIONS AND SYMBOLS*

Capacity	Temperature
Cup (c)	Degrees Celsius (°C)
Deciliter (d)	Degrees Fahrenheit (°F)
Fluid ounce (fl oz)	**Length**
Gallon (gal)	Centimeter (cm)
Liter (l)	Foot (ft)
Milliliter (ml)	Inch (in)
Pint (pt)	Meter (m)
Quart (qt)	Millimeter (mm)
Peck (pk)	Millimicron (mμ)
Bushel (bu)	**Weight**
Gill (gi)	Gram (g)
Tablespoon (Tbsp)	Kilogram (kg)
Teaspoon (tsp)	Microgram (μg)
Time	Milligram (mg)
Hour (hr)	Ounce (oz)
Minute (min)	Pound (lb)
Second (sec)	

*Note that abbreviations are used in the singular form regardless of whether the item is singular or plural. For metric units, a symbol is used, such as g for grams.

WEIGHT AND VOLUME EQUIVALENTS

Common Units of Weight		
1 gram	=	0.035 ounces
1 kilogram	=	2.21 pounds
1 ounce	=	28.35 grams
1 pound	=	453.59 grams
Common Units of Volume		
1 bushel	=	4 pecks
1 peck	=	8 quarts
1 gallon	=	4 quarts
1 quart	=	2 pints
		946.4 milliliters
1 pint	=	2 cups
1 cup	=	16 tablespoons
		2 gills
		8 fluid ounces
		236.6 milliliters
1 Tablespoon	=	3 teaspoons
		½ fluid ounce
		14.8 milliliters
1 teaspoon	=	4.9 milliliters
1 liter	=	1000 milliliters
		1.06 quarts
1 dash	=	1/8 teaspoon
1 pinch	=	1/16 teaspoon
1 smidgen	=	1/32 teaspoon

TABLE OF EQUIVALENTS (CONTINUED)
EQUIVALENTS FOR ONE UNIT AND FRACTIONS OF A UNIT

Tablespoon		
1 Tbsp	=	3 tsp
⅞ Tbsp	=	2½ tsp
¾ Tbsp	=	2¼ tsp
⅔ Tbsp	=	2 tsp
⅝ Tbsp	=	1⅞ tsp
½ Tbsp	=	1½ tsp
⅜ Tbsp	=	1⅛ tsp
⅓ Tbsp	=	1 tsp
¼ Tbsp	=	¾ tsp

Cup		
1 c	=	16 Tbsp
⅞ c	=	14 Tbsp
¾ c	=	12 Tbsp
⅔ c	=	10⅔ Tbsp
⅝ c	=	10 Tbsp
½ c	=	8 Tbsp
⅜ c	=	6 Tbsp
⅓ c	=	5⅓ Tbsp
¼ c	=	4 Tbsp
⅛ c	=	2 Tbsp
1⁄16 c	=	1 Tbsp

Pint		
1 pt	=	2 c
⅞ pt	=	1¾ c
¾ pt	=	1½ c
⅔ pt	=	1⅓ c
⅝ pt	=	1¼ c
½ pt	=	1 c
⅜ pt	=	¾ c
⅓ pt	=	⅔ c
¼ pt	=	½ c
⅛ pt	=	¼ c
1⁄16 pt	=	2 Tbsp

Quart		
1 qt	=	2 pt
⅞ qt	=	3½ c
¾ qt	=	3 c
⅔ qt	=	2⅔ c
⅝ qt	=	2½ c
½ qt	=	1 pt
⅜ qt	=	1½ c
⅓ qt	=	1⅓ c
¼ qt	=	1 c
⅛ qt	=	½ c
1⁄16 qt	=	¼ c

Gallon		
1 gal	=	4 qt
⅞ gal	=	3½ qt
¾ gal	=	3 qt
⅔ gal	=	10⅔ c
⅝ gal	=	5 pt
½ gal	=	2 qt
⅜ gal	=	3 pt
⅓ gal	=	5⅓ c
¼ gal	=	1 qt
⅛ gal	=	1 pt
1⁄16 gal	=	1 c

Pound		
1 lb	=	16 oz
⅞ lb	=	14 oz
¾ lb	=	12 oz
⅔ lb	=	10⅔ oz
⅝ lb	=	10 oz
½ lb	=	8 oz
⅜ lb	=	6 oz
⅓ lb	=	5⅓ oz
¼ lb	=	4 oz
⅛ lb	=	2 oz
1⁄16 lb	=	1 oz

TABLE 1.2
COOKING CONVERSIONS

U.S. TO METRIC

Capacity	
⅕ teaspoon	1 milliliter
1 teaspoon	5 milliliters
1 tablespoon	15 milliliters
1 fluid ounce	30 milliliters
⅕ cup	47 milliliters
1 cup	237 milliliters
2 cups (1 pint)	473 milliliters
4 cups (1 quart)	0.95 liter
4 quarts (1 gallon)	3.8 liters
Weight	
1 ounce	28 grams
1 pound	454 grams

METRIC TO U.S.

Capacity	
1 milliliter	⅕ teaspoon
5 milliliters	1 teaspoon
15 milliliters	1 tablespoon
100 milliliters	3.4 fluid ounces
240 milliliters	1 cup
1 liter	34 fluid ounces
	4.2 cups
	2.1 pints
	1.06 quarts
	0.26 gallon
Weight	
1 gram	0.035 ounce
100 grams	3.5 ounces
500 grams	1.10 pounds
1 kilogram	2.205 pounds
	35 ounces

RECIPE FORMS

Recipes may be printed in various forms. The most common are Standard, Descriptive, Action, and Narrative. The Standard form lists ingredients at the top followed by the methods. The Descriptive form displays ingredients, amounts, and procedures in three columns left to right. Ingredients, amounts, and procedures also are separated horizontally into groups that follow the sequence of the recipe. The Action form recipe lists procedures in sequence with each procedure accompanied by the ingredients needed for that procedure. In Narrative form, the recipe is written in a paragraph with sentences that include ingredients, amounts, and preparation methods.

When an ingredient has modifications, the exact specification can make a difference, For example: 2 cups sifted flour (sifted and then measured) is not the same as 2 cups flour, sifted (measured and then sifted). If cream is to be in liquid form, then the recipe may state, 1 cup heavy whipped cream (measured in a liquid measuring cup). This is different from 1 cup heavy cream, whipped (measured in a dry measuring cup).

Standard Form

Blueberry Muffins

¾ cup milk
¼ cup vegetable oil
1 large egg
1⅓ cup all-purpose flour
⅔ cup whole wheat flour
½ cup sugar
2 teaspoons baking powder
½ teaspoon salt
1 cup fresh or frozen blueberries

Preheat oven to 400°F. Spray bottom of 12 medium muffin cups with cooking spray or line with paper baking cups.

In large bowl, beat milk, oil, and egg with fork or whisk until well mixed. Add flour, sugar, baking powder, and salt all at once, stirring only until flour is moistened (batter will be lumpy). Fold in blueberries. Portion batter evenly among muffin cups.

Bake 20 to 25 minutes until golden brown. Remove muffins from pan to cool on a rack.

Descriptive Form

Blueberry Muffins

Portions: 12 muffins
Oven temperature: 400°F

Ingredients	Amount	Procedure
Milk	¾ cup	In large bowl, beat milk, oil, and egg with fork or whisk until well mixed.
Vegetable oil	¼ cup	
Egg, large	1	
Flour, all-purpose	1⅓ cup	Add dry ingredients to liquid mixture all at once. Stir just until flour is moistened (batter will be lumpy).
Flour, whole wheat	⅔ cup	
Sugar	½ cup	
Baking powder	2 tsp	
Salt	½ tsp	
Blueberries fresh or frozen	1 cup	Fold in blueberries.
		Portion batter into muffin cups. Bake 20 to 25 minutes until golden brown. Remove muffins to a rack for cooling.

Action Form

Blueberry Muffins

Preheat oven to 400°F. Spray 12 muffin cups with cooking spray or line with paper baking cups.

Measure into mixing bowl and beat with fork or whisk until well mixed:
   ¾ cup milk
   ¼ cup vegetable oil
   1 large egg

Add following ingredients to liquid mixture:
1⅓ cup all-purpose flour
⅔ cup whole wheat flour
½ cup sugar
2 teaspoons baking powder
½ teaspoon salt

Stir until flour is moistened (batter will be lumpy).

Fold in: 1 cup blueberries (fresh or frozen)

Portion batter evenly among muffin cups.

Bake 20 to 25 minutes or until golden brown.

Remove muffins from pan to cool on a rack.

Narrative Form

Blueberry Muffins

Preheat oven to 400°F. Spray 12 muffin cups with cooking spray or line with paper baking cups. In large bowl beat ¾ cup milk, ¼ cup vegetable oil, and 1 large egg with fork or whisk until well mixed. Then add the following dry ingredients all at once: 1⅓ cup all-purpose flour, ⅔ cup whole wheat flour, ½ cup sugar, 2 teaspoons baking powder, and ½ teaspoon salt. Stir only until flour is moistened (batter will be lumpy). Fold in 1 cup blueberries (fresh or frozen). Portion batter evenly among muffin cups. Bake 20 to 25 minutes or until golden brown. Remove muffins from pan to cool on a rack.

INGREDIENTS

1. List all ingredients with measurements in the order used.

2. Use standard abbreviations and measurements (Table 1:1).

3. Provide ingredients in the fewest number of units of measure, such as ¼ cup instead of 4 tablespoons. Use standard abbreviations and measurements (Table 1:1).

4. Use weights instead of measures when it is helpful, as for uncooked meat, poultry, fish, cheese, and similar foods. Include weight or fluid measure for canned products.

5. Specify types of products needed, such as cake flour, all-purpose flour, dark corn syrup.

6. For eggs, list egg yolks or egg whites or eggs, and include simple preparation, such as eggs, slightly beaten. If special preparation is needed, such as for meringue, explain in the method, detailing all necessary steps.

7. If possible, give the generic terms for products used.

METHOD

1. Use short sentences and clear, simple directions that anyone can follow easily.

2. Give word pictures, like chill until syrupy, or beat until foamy throughout, or mixture thickens as it cools. These are helpful, particularly with unfamiliar mixtures.

3. Use methods for combining or cooking ingredients that represent best accepted procedures. For example, specify the best way to sift dry ingredients together, or to thicken a sauce, or to fold in beaten egg white—these can be expressed in the same terms whenever they occur in recipes. This practice results in a standardized consistency of phrasing from recipe to recipe.

4. Give thought to the most efficient order of work to avoid using extra bowls, cups, measuring tools, extra beating, and so forth.

5. Specify standard sizes of baking pans or casseroles, such as: 9-inch round layer pans, 1½ inches deep or shallow 1-quart casserole.

6. Try to provide both general and specific tests or temperatures. Then the recipe provides a double check on important stages. For example: Cook to 238°F or until a small amount of syrup forms a soft ball in cold water.

7. For the yield, give the number and size of servings to expect or the total measure, such as: Makes 4, 1-cup servings or 1 quart.

ACCURACY

1. Read over the edited recipe. Does it say exactly what is meant? Is it simple, clear, and complete, yet as brief as it can be?

2. Recheck the ingredients, amounts, and method against the original recipe data. Recheck the order of ingredients as listed against the order used. Check for any omissions in temperatures, times, yields, etc. Tell whether a canned ingredient should be drained or a pan covered during cooking.

3. With every production of the recipe, read the new copy carefully against the former copy.

4. With every printing of the recipe, check first proofs against original correct copy, then proofread at each succeeding stage. Read proofs just for sense at least once.

OVEN TEMPERATURE TERMINOLOGY

In giving oven temperatures, most recipe writers state the degrees first and follow with the descriptive term, thus, 400°F or 200°C (hot) oven. The following listing shows the commonly accepted descriptive terms for each temperature range in degrees Fahrenheit and Celsius

Fahrenheit	Celsius	Descriptor
250° to 275°	120° to 140°	Lukewarm oven
300° to 325°	150° to 160°	Warm oven
350° to 375°	180° to 190°	Moderate oven
400° to 425°	200° to 220°	Hot oven
450° to 475°	230° to 240°	Very hot oven
500° to 525°	260° to 270°	Extremely hot oven

MODIFICATION OF RECIPES TO MEET DIETARY GUIDELINES

Because the link between diet and health is so important, the U.S. Department of Agriculture (USDA) and the U.S. Department of Health and Human Services (HHS) periodically update and release Dietary Guidelines for Americans to help people make wise dietary decisions in order to eat for health. In 2011, the USDA introduced ChooseMyPlate as a simple guide to healthy food consumption for consumers. ChooseMyPlate replaces the 1992 Food Pyramid and shows a simple circle representing a plate divided into four quadrants. Half of the plate contains fruits and vegetables. Whole grains occupy another quarter of the plate while lean proteins (legumes, fish, lean meat, and poultry) take up the remaining quarter. Skim or 1% milk and dairy and calcium-fortified soy products are represented by a glass of milk to the side of the plate. For more information, visit www.choosemyplate.gov.

Key messages of the 2010 Dietary Guidelines:

- **Balance Calories**
  Individuals are encouraged to balance calories consumed and calories expended by watching what, when, why, and how much is eaten.

- **Be Active Your Way**
  Individuals are encouraged to balance healthy eating with regular physical activity.

Foods to Reduce	Foods to Increase
Sodium	Variety of foods within caloric needs
Solid fats	Vegetables
Saturated fats	Fruits
Trans fatty acids	Whole Grains
Added sugars	Milk and milk products*
Refined grains	Lean meats, poultry, fish, eggs, beans, and nuts**

* Fat-free and low fat milk products
**To increase potassium, dietary fiber, calcium, and vitamin D

Most people can benefit by modifying what foods they choose to eat. However, another way to modify diet is to make adjustments in the types and amounts of ingredients in recipes to produce more nutrient dense food products (i.e., lower in fat or salt, higher in fiber).

WHEN TO MODIFY RECIPES

Not all recipes need to be modified. Consider the following questions.

1. **Is the recipe already low in fat, cholesterol, sugar, or salt?** If so, only minor or no changes may be needed. For example, if a recipe calls for an egg, and the dish serves eight people, the amount of cholesterol per serving already is low.

2. **How often is the food eaten?** It is not as important to modify a recipe for a dish eaten once or twice a year as it is for food eaten frequently. For example, it is more important to cut the fat in a weekly sub sandwich or salad than it is to cut the fat in an annual birthday cake.

3. **How much of the food is eaten?** Sometimes the best way to modify the intake of a certain food is to eat less of it. Decreasing the quantity eaten may be more satisfying than altering the recipe to contain less fat or kilocalories.

HOW TO MODIFY RECIPES

1. **Identify the dietary goal and decide which nutrients to modify.** To reduce kilocalories (also known as food calories [1000 calories] and in this book referred to only as calories, Cal, kcal) (1 kcal=4.18 kilojoules or kJ), identify ingredients that contribute the most calories (or kilojoules), usually fat and/or alcohol, and reduce or remove and substitute those ingredients. To reduce sodium or sugar, and to increase fiber, identify ingredients containing these components and lower/increase the amounts or use substitutions.

    Kilocalories: Fat is the most concentrated source of kilocalories (9 kcal / 38 kJ) followed by alcohol (7 kcal / 30 kJ) as compared to protein and carbohydrates (4 kcal/ 17 kJ). Reducing the amount of fat in a recipe is the most effective way to cut calories.

    Fat: Fatty acids are basic components of fat. They can be classified as saturated, trans, monounsaturated, or polyunsaturated. All fats in foods contain mixtures of these fatty acids. Consumption of high amounts of saturated fats and trans fats raises the level of serum cholesterol and increases risk of cardiovascular disease for individuals.

    Saturated fats are found in the largest proportions in fats of animal origin such as whole milk, cream, cheese, butter, lard, meat, and poultry. They also occur in large amounts in coconut oil and palm kernel oil.

    Trans fatty acids are formed when oils are partially hydrogenated to produce more solid fats such as margarine or hydrogenated shortening. This process increases shelf life, flavor stability, and melting point for these fats. Trans fats are found mainly in processed foods made with partially hydrogenated shortening or margarine including crackers, cookies, cakes, pies, snack foods, and other baked foods.

Foods that are fried in partially hydrogenated shortening such as French fried potatoes are also high in trans fat content. Because these fats increase low-density lipoprotein (LDL, "bad") cholesterol and decrease high-density lipoproteins (HDL, "good") cholesterol, read and use food labels (changed in 2006 to include trans-fat information) to decrease trans fatty acid intake.

Monounsaturated fats are found in large amounts in canola oil, olive oil, and peanut oil, as well as in many margarines and semi-solid vegetable shortenings.

Polyunsaturated fats are found in the largest proportions in fats of plant origin such as liquid vegetable oils (safflower, sunflower, corn, cottonseed, and soybean) and margarines and salad dressings made from them.

Omega-3 fatty acids help to reduce inflammation, blood pressure, blood clotting, and triglycerides (a fat-like substance) in the blood. Seek ways to promote healthy omega-3 fatty acid intakes by increasing consumption of walnuts, flax seeds, olive oil, soybean oil, and fatty fish (salmon, trout, Atlantic and Pacific mackerel, herring, tuna (fresh and canned), and sardines.

Cholesterol is a fat-like substance found only in food of animal origin. Sources include egg yolks, meats (particularly organ meats), butter, cream, and cheese.

Sugar comes in many forms, for example, white sugar, brown sugar, raw sugar, honey, corn syrup, molasses, and maple syrup.

Sodium is present in salt (salt is 40 percent sodium), baking soda, baking powder, monosodium glutamate (MSG), soy sauce, bouillon, pickles, olives, cured meats, many canned vegetables and convenience foods, most cheeses, sauces, and soups.

Fiber is present in whole grain breads and cereals; dry beans and peas; nuts and seeds; and fruits and vegetables, especially those with edible skins or seeds.

2. **Determine how to change the ingredient(s) to achieve the dietary goal**. Ingredient(s) can be:

a. eliminated completely

b. reduced in amount

c. substituted for a more nutritionally acceptable ingredient

To choose the best approach, it is helpful to have a general idea of the function of the ingredients, and what will happen if they are modified. Table 1.3 lists the function and nutritional contribution of several ingredients.

TIPS FOR HEALTHY MODIFICATIONS

The following are a few ways to modify recipes. These suggestions can be applied to most food; exceptions include those in which specific proportions of ingredients are essential to prevent spoilage or to create a certain product consistency (such as salt in cured meats or pickles, or sugar in jams and jellies).

1. To Decrease Total Fat and Kilocalories

- Reduce fat by one-fourth to one-third in baked products. For example, if a recipe calls for 1 cup (250 ml) shortening, try ⅔ cup (165 ml). This works satisfactorily in many quick breads, muffins, and cookies.

- Replace one-third to one-half of fat in baked products by substituting bananas, applesauce, or prune puree.

- Sauté or stir-fry vegetables with little fat or simmer in water, wine, or broth.

- Steam or microwave vegetables.

- To thicken sauces and gravies without lumping, eliminate fat and instead mix cornstarch or flour with double the measured amount of cold liquid. Stir this mixture slowly into the hot liquid to be thickened and bring it to a boil, stirring constantly.

- Add herbs, spices, or flavorings.

- Chill soups, gravies, and stews, and skim off hardened fat before reheating to serve.

- Select lean cuts of meat and trim off visible fat. Remove skin from poultry before cooking.

- Bake, broil, grill, poach, or microwave meat, poultry, or fish instead of frying in fat.

- Decrease the proportion of oil in homemade salad dressings. Try one-third oil to two-thirds vinegar. Low-fat cottage cheese, yogurt, and buttermilk seasoned with herbs and spices also make low-fat dressings.

- Use reduced-calorie or nonfat sour cream, mayonnaise, plain low-fat or nonfat yogurt, buttermilk, or blended cottage cheese instead of regular sour cream or mayonnaise for sauces, dips, and salad dressings. If a sauce made with yogurt is to be heated, blend one tablespoon of cornstarch with one cup of yogurt to prevent separation.

- Use nonfat or low-fat milk instead of whole milk. For extra richness, add undiluted evaporated skim milk.

- Choose low-fat cheeses such as feta, Neufchatel, and mozzarella instead of high-fat ones such as Swiss or Cheddar. Also use less cheese.

2. To Decrease Saturated Fat and Cholesterol

- Use two egg whites or an egg substitute product instead of one whole egg. In some recipes, simply decrease the total number of eggs. This is especially true if the fat is also decreased in the recipe.

- Use olive oil on breads/toast instead of margarine or butter. Otherwise, look for margarines in which liquid vegetable oil is the first ingredient listed on the label.

- Use vegetable oils instead of solid fats. To substitute liquid oil for solid fats, use about one-fourth less than the recipe calls for. For example, if a recipe calls for ¼ cup or 4 tablespoons (60 ml) of solid fat, use 3 tablespoons (45 ml) of oil. For cakes or piecrusts, use a recipe that specifically calls for oil because liquid fats require special mixing procedures.

3. To Decrease Sugar

- Reduce sugar by one-quarter to one-third in some baked goods and desserts. Add extra spice or flavoring to enhance impression of sweetness. This works best with quick breads, cookies, pie fillings, custard, puddings, and fruit crisps.

- Decrease or eliminate sugar when canning or freezing fruits. Buy unsweetened frozen fruit or fruit canned in its own juice or water.

- In cookies, bar and drop, replace one-quarter of sugar called for with an equal proportion of nonfat dry milk; this reduces kilocalories and increases calcium, protein, and riboflavin in the recipe.

- Choose fruit juices, club soda, or skim milk over soft drinks and punches. Make fruit juice coolers with equal parts fruit juice and club soda or seltzer.

- Nonsugar sweeteners now on the market include aspartame, acesulfame potassium, saccharin, stevia, and sucralose. All of these sugar substitutes work well in some applications, but aspartame and saccharin are not recommended for use in baked products. Both acesulfame postassium and and sucralose are marketed in sugar blends for baking that produce acceptable results with a small reduction in calories. The beginning cook is advised to use recipes especially developed for these products.

4. To Decrease Sodium

- Salt may be omitted or reduced in most recipes. Do not reduce the salt in cured meats or pickled or brined vegetables, because it acts as a preservative. A small amount is also useful in yeast breads to help control the rising action of the yeast.

- Start with a gradual reduction. For example, if a recipe calls for 1 teaspoon (5 ml) of salt, try ½ teaspoon (2 ml). If the amount of salt is reduced gradually, an individual will soon adjust taste references to foods containing less salt.

- Choose fresh or low-sodium versions of products. For example, choose low-sodium soups and broths, soy sauce, canned vegetables, and tomato products.

- Rely on herbs and spices rather than salt for flavor.

- Use garlic or onion powder instead of garlic or onion salt.

- Reduce the salt used in cooking pasta, noodles, rice or hot cereals.

- Use water from the cold water tap for cooking. Water softeners contain sodium, but the amount of sodium differs according to the hardness of the untreated water. Untreated water is best used for cooking and softened water can be used for hot water needs and cleaning.

- Dilute broth or bouillon with water when using as the cooking liquid.

- Read labels. Any ingredient with "sodium" as part of the name includes sodium. The amount of sodium per serving is listed in the Nutrition Facts section of food labels.

5. To Increase Fiber

- Choose whole grain instead of highly refined products (e.g., whole-wheat flour and bread, bulgur, brown rice, oatmeal, whole-corn meal, and barley).

- Whole-wheat flour usually can be substituted for up to one-half of the all-purpose refined flour in a recipe. For example, if a recipe calls for 2 cups (500 ml) of all-purpose flour, try 1 cup (250 ml) of all-purpose and 1 cup (250 ml) of whole-wheat flour.

- Add extra fruits and vegetables to recipes and substitute fruit and vegetable purees for some ingredients.

- Add fruits to muffins, pancakes, salads, and desserts, and add vegetables to quiche fillings, casseroles, and salads.

6. To Increase Food Safety

- Specify pasteurized eggs or egg substitutes for recipes with raw or undercooked eggs (meringues, homemade ice creams, etc.).

- Promote use of accurate temperature checks using an appropriate and calibrated thermometer.

- Update and correct food temperatures since the requirements change as research reveals necessary corrections. For most current food safety changes, check on the USDA or AAFCS websites.

PUTTING IT INTO PRACTICE

To begin, look at the ingredients in the recipe and review their functions (Table 1.3). Then look at the general guidelines for modifying ingredients. Use the following steps when modifying a baked product.

1. Compare the recipe with the basic recipe proportions given in this book. To do this, express ingredients in terms of 1 cup of flour (250 ml). For example, if the recipe calls for 2 cups of flour (500 ml) and ½ cup sugar (125 ml), it calls for ¼ cup sugar (60 ml) for every 1 cup flour (250 ml).

2. Decide which ingredients to reduce. Compare the amounts of fat, eggs, sugar, and salt per 1 cup (250 ml) flour with amounts given in a basic recipe proportion table. Those on the high end of the range are the ones to reduce. Reduce fat and/or sugar to at least the midpoint of the range.

Reduce eggs, if needed, to within range. Reduce sodium if desired.

3. Decide which ingredients to increase. Fat and sugar provide moistness and richness to recipes. When they are reduced, liquid needs to be added, usually in the form of water, milk, fruit juice, applesauce, or fruit or vegetable pulp. Fruit and vegetable pulp also add fiber; milk adds calcium. Add back at least half as much liquid as the volume of reduced sugar and fat reduced. For example, if the sugar is reduced in a recipe by 2 tablespoons (30 ml) and fat by 4 tablespoons (60 ml), add 3 tablespoons (45 ml) milk or fruit juice. Because honey and molasses have greater moisture retaining properties than sugar, replacing a portion of the sugar that remains in the recipe with honey or molasses may improve softness and moistness in the end product.

4. Consider adding nonfat dry milk to increase calcium content. In many baked products, nonfat dry milk can replace up to one-fourth of the sugar in the recipe with good results. Two to four tablespoons (30 to 60 ml) of nonfat dry milk powder per cup (250 ml) of flour also may be added to cookies and cakes as an additive. Look at the recipe and add nonfat dry milk powder equal to the reduction in sugar.

5. Try recipe with modifications made. Use the toothpick or touch test, not just visual appearance, to evaluate doneness. Because sugar slows protein coagulation and slows starch gelatinization, products made with reduced sugar will bake more quickly and be less brown when done.

6. Evaluate the quality and taste of the product. If the recipe still seems richer than desired, make further reductions in fat and sugar and increase liquid. If the product seems dry, be careful to not over bake. If still dry and not over-baked, try adding more liquid (water, fruit juice, applesauce, fruit, or vegetable pulp), or substitute a portion of the sugar in the recipe with honey or molasses.

7. Try reformulated recipe and repeat steps 5 and 6 until pleased with results. Remember to record the modifications that work. Recipes that meet the Dietary Guidelines are worth repeating. The Carrot Bread recipe (on page 15) is an example of an original recipe with modifications.

TABLE 1.3
FUNCTION AND NUTRITIONAL CONTRIBUTION OF BAKING INGREDIENTS

Ingredient	Function	Kilocalories (Kilojules)	Nutritional Value
Flour	Contributes structure and rigidity. Gives stretch or elasticity. Provides thickening.	460/cup (1925)	Provides complex carbohydrates, some protein, source of B vitamins, and iron if enriched or whole grain.
Liquid	Dissolves dry ingredients (flour, sugar, salt). Moistens flour to develop structure. Dissolves leavening agents, e.g., baking powder, baking soda.	Water = 0/cup Milk = 80-160/cup (335-670)	Milk is a good source of calcium, riboflavin, protein; also provides vitamin A, B12, and phosphorus. Whole milk contains some saturated fat.

FUNCTION AND NUTRITIONAL CONTRIBUTION OF BAKING INGREDIENTS (CONTINUED)

Ingredient	Function	Kilocalories (Kilojules)	Nutritional Value
Salt	Helps improve taste. Prevents large air cells in yeast products by controlling rising.	0 units	Provides 2,000 mg sodium / tsp (5 ml) and 3,000 mg chloride.
Leavening Agents	Important for structure and lightness.	0 units	Baking powder and soda contain sodium; yeast does not.
Sugar	Adds sweetness. Increases volume. Helps tenderize product. Aids in browning.	Sugar = 770 / cup (3222) Honey = 1020 / cup (4269) Molasses = 700-825 / cup (2930-3453)	Provides energy. Molasses provides some calcium and iron.
Fat	Helps tenderize. Adds flavor to product. Increases moistness.	Lard, shortening, oil = 135 / Tbsp (520), 2160 / cup (8032) Butter / Margarine = 110 / Tbsp 1760 / cup (460-7366)	Provides fat calories and fat soluble vitamins. Butter, lard, vegetable shortening and palm and coconut oil are higher in saturated than polyunsaturated fat. Soft margarine and other oils are higher in polyunsaturated fat. Butter, lard, and other animal fats contain cholesterol. Butter and margarine provide some sodium and vitamin A. Vegetable oils provide vitamin E.
Eggs	Contribute to elasticity and structure. Beaten whites incorporate air into batters. Yolks add color and emulsify fats.	80 / egg (335)	Provide protein and small amounts of several nutrients. Egg yolk rich in fat, saturated fat, and cholesterol.
Nuts	Flavor and variety.	750-850 / cup (3139-3557)	Provide some protein, B vitamins, iron, and fiber. Generally rich in fat and polyunsaturated fat.
Fruits and Vegetables	Flavor and variety.	Fruits = 100-200 / cup (418-837) Vegetables = 20-150 / cup (84-628)	Generally good source of B vitamins and vitamins A and/or C. Good source of fiber, especially when skins and tiny seeds are consumed.

CARROT BREAD

Original Recipe	Kcal/(kJ)	Modified Recipe	Kcal/(kJ)	Improvement(s) Made
Sugar, ¾ cup (175 ml)	578 (2419)	Sugar, ¼ cup (60 ml)	192 (804)	Decreased sugar
		Orange juice, ½ cup (125 ml)	60 (251)	Increased vitamin C, folic acid, and moisture
Soybean oil, 1 cup (250 ml)	1920 (8035)	Corn oil, ⅓ cup (80 ml)	636 (2662)	Decreased fat, kilocalories
Eggs, 2	160 (670)	Egg, 1	80 (335)	Decreased cholesterol
Vanilla, 1½ tsp (7 ml)	0	Same	0	
All-purpose flour, 2 cups (500 ml)	910 (3808)	All-purpose flour 1 cup (250 ml)	862 (3607)	Increased fiber and trace minerals
		Whole wheat flour 1 cup (250 ml)		
Baking Powder, 1 tsp (5 ml)	0	Same	0	
Baking Soda, ½ tsp (2 ml)	0	Same	0	
Cinnamon, 1 Tbsp (15 ml)	0	Same	0	
Salt, ½ tsp (2 ml)	0	Salt, ¼ tsp (1 ml)	0	Decreased sodium
Carrots, grated 1¼ cups (300 ml)	50 (209)	Carrots, grated 1½ cups (375 ml)	60 (251)	Increased vitamin A, beta-carotene, and fiber
TOTALS: Recipe	3618 (15141)		1890 (7910)	
½-inch slice (1.25 cm)	201 (841)		105 (439)	

Directions: Beat together sugar, oil, eggs, orange juice, and vanilla. Stir dry ingredients together and add to sugar and oil mixture. Blend in grated carrots. Bake in oiled 9 x 5-inch (23 x 13 cm) loaf pan at 350°F (180°C) for 40 to 50 minutes.

HIGH-ALTITUDE FOOD PREPARATION

At altitudes above 3000 feet (914 m), food preparation by traditional, microwave, or campfire methods may require changes in time, temperature, recipe proportions, microwave power levels, and/or pan size. The reason is reduced atmospheric pressure at higher elevations; the pressure decreases about ½ pound per 1000 feet or 2.2 Newtons per 305 meters increase in elevation. Pressure per square inch (0.645 square meters) at sea level is 14.7 pounds (6.7 kg), at 5000 feet (1524 m) is 12.3 pounds (5.6 kg), and at 10,000 feet (3048 m) is 10.2 pounds (4.6 kg). This decreased pressure affects food preparation in several ways:

- Water and liquids boil at lower temperatures and evaporate faster.

- Leavening gases in breads and cakes expand more.

- Liquids foam more quickly, and cakes and breads rise more during baking; liquid or cakes may flow over the sides of the pan.

- Microwaved foods thaw and reheat at a slightly slower rate.

- Foods microwaved at 5000 feet (1524 m) versus sea level are often more moist, but they cool and dry out rapidly. Store baked goods covered.

- Foods cook more slowly in boiling water as altitude increases.

- Approximate boiling temperatures of water at various elevations:

Sea level	212.0°F/100.0°C
2000 feet / 610 meters	208.2°F / 97.8°C
5000 feet / 1524 meters	202.5°F / 94.5°C
7500 feet / 2286 meters	197.8°F / 91.8°C
10,000 feet / 3048 meters	193.0°F / 89.0°C

Each 1000 feet (304.8 m) increase in elevation decreases the boiling point temperature 1.9°F (1.1°C).

BOILED, COOKED, AND FRIED FOODS GUIDELINES

Because water boils at lower temperatures at higher altitudes, food products require a longer cooking time to reach the desired end point.

Beverages/Soups: Increase the amount of coffee/tea and brew time for similar flavors. Brew in pot rather than cup to release flavors and maintain heat. Above 8000 feet (2438 m), brewed beverages are not very hot. Homemade soups need more time and water. Milk-based beverages boil over easily.

Vegetables: Increase boiling time 4–11 percent at 5000 feet (1524 m), 20–25 percent at 7200 feet (2194 m), and 55–66 percent at 10,000 feet (3048 m) and add more water. Foil-wrapped potatoes with roast at 325°F (160°C) need 2–2½ hours at 5000 (1524 m) and 7500 feet (2286 m), and 3 hours at 10,000 feet (3048 m). Prick potatoes to prevent explosions during baking. A general rule for microwaving fresh whole vegetables is to heat on high for 7 minutes/pound (454g) for cut vegetables, then add 1–2 tablespoons (15–30 ml) water and microwave ½–1 minute more. For frozen vegetables, add 2–4 tablespoons (30–60 ml) water and 1–3 minutes more time. To prepare dried beans, soak overnight, and then cook, using 2–3 times more water and greatly increased time; a pressure saucepan is recommended for cooking soaked, dried beans at altitudes above 7500 feet (2286 m).

Meat/Poultry: For moist-heat cooking at 5000 feet (1524 m) 25–50 percent more time is needed for braising or simmering meat and 5 to 35 minutes more time for microwaving. Watch the liquid levels, and use tight fitting lids. Microwave for the first period on High for 8–10 minutes until boiling, then cook at lower power until fork tender. For dry heat roasting in a hot oven, use the same or slightly longer cooking times; check for doneness with a thermometer. Large or dense pieces may need 10–25 percent more time. A three-pound (1.36 kg) chicken needs 10–15 minutes more roasting time or 3–5 minutes more when microwaving. Pan-fry at slightly higher settings; increase electric skillet/wok temperature by 25°F (14°C). For grilling, a partial precook and frequent basting are helpful to prevent drying of meat. NOTE: Charcoal briquettes need 45 minutes to become 70 percent ashed-over at 5000 feet (1524 m) versus 20–25 minutes at sea level. In the microwave, one pound (454 g) ground meat needs 1–3 minutes more time.

Fruits and steamed puddings: More time for all cooking methods may be needed. Above 7500 feet (2286 m), precooking pie fruit is desirable.

Egg cooking:

Altitude	Soft cooked	Hard cooked
5000 feet / 1524 meters	5–6 minutes	20–25 minutes
7500 feet / 2286 meters	7 minutes	23–27 minutes
10,000 feet / 3048 meters	9 minutes	26 minutes

Slight time increases are needed for poached eggs.

Sugar cooking: Candies, syrups, frostings, and jellies need a decrease in the final cooked-stage temperature. The temperature should be decreased by the difference in the boiling water temperature at the preparation altitude and that of sea level. Example: A thermometer in boiling water reads 202°F (94.5°C) or ten degrees below 212°F (5.5 below 100°C). For soft-ball candy, subtract 10 degrees from 238°F (114°C) and cook only to 228°F (5.5 from 114.5°C or 109°C). The cold water candy and jelly sheeting tests are the same as at sea level. Microwaved candies foam up more, so use a larger dish or make half of the recipe.

Starch cooking: At altitudes of 5000 feet (1524 m) or higher, problems may be encountered in the use of cornstarch for thickening. Direct heat, a heavy saucepan (not a double boiler) and constant stirring to prevent scorching are needed for the starch to reach maximum gelatinization. Above 7500 feet (2286 m), replace 1 tablespoon (15 ml) of cornstarch with 2 tablespoons (30 ml) flour in pudding/filling. When microwaving, make sure the whole mixture is boiling and thickened; add time if necessary.

Rice/Pasta: Add 1 teaspoon (5 ml) oil per cup of rice/pasta to prevent sticking and boiling over. For rice at 5000 feet (1524 m) add an additional 4–8 tablespoons (60-120 ml) water per 1 cup (236.6 ml) of water in the recipe and increase time by 25–30 percent. When microwaving, cook on high 5–8 minutes until boiling and continue at 50-percent power, increase time by 30–40 percent. For pasta, keep water at an adequate boil, taste test, and generally add more cooking time. When microwaving cereals use a large bowl. In casseroles with rice, pasta, dried beans, and firm vegetables, precook these items. For milk-based casseroles, use a larger dish to prevent boiling over.

Deep-fat frying: The lower boiling point of water in foods requires lowering the temperature of the fat to prevent overbrowned but raw foods. A rough guide is to lower the frying temperature about 2–3°F for each 1000 feet (1 to 1.5°C per 304.8 m) increase in elevation. Example: At 8000 feet (2438 m), doughnuts need frying fat temperatures at 359°F to 351°F for 24 to 16°F (183 to 177°C or 13 to 7°C) lower. Cake-like doughnuts may need less baking powder, sugar, and/or shortening.

Canning, pressure canning, and refreezing: See Chapter 13, Food Preservation. Pressure saucepans designed only for pressure-cooking should not be used for canning.

Pressure saucepans: Pans that are designed ONLY for pressure cooking and NOT canning require an increase in pressure to achieve the required processing temperature.

STEAM PRESSURES AT VARIOUS ALTITUDES

Altitude		Pressure Required for 240°F, 116°C		Pressure Required for 250°F, 121°C	
Feet	Meters	lb	kPa	lb	kPa
Sea Level	0	10	68.9	15	103.4
1000	305	10.5	72.4	15.5	106.8
2000	610	11	75.8	16	110.3
3000	914	11.5	79.3	16.5	113.8
4000	1219	12	82.7	17	117.2
5000	1524	12.5	86.2	17.5	120.7
7000	2134	13.5	93.1	18.5	127.6
10000	3048	15	103.4	20	137.9

LEAVENED AND BAKED FOODS GUIDELINES

Because the atmospheric pressure is less at higher elevations, leavened baked products can rise excessively, stretching the cell structure, producing a coarse, irregular texture, overflowing the pan sides, and even falling in the center with a sway or depression and low volume. Quick breads, if low in sugar, are firm enough to withstand the excess rising and need only to have leavening reduced, liquid added, and temperature and maybe pan size increased. For cookies, see "Hints" on page 19. Generally, microwaved cakes require fewer adjustments than do cakes baked in an oven. Most cakes, cake-like products, and breads are affected slightly at 2000 feet (610 m) and significantly above 3500 feet (1067 m). Adjustments in the recipe are needed above 3500 feet (1067 m). There are no "formulas" for adjusting and only repeated tests can determine the most successful adjusted recipe.

Recipe adjustments to improve baked products: This includes cake, quick breads, cookies, bar cookies, brownies, pancakes, and doughnuts. Try the lower range when a range is given.

Oven temperature — Increase 15 to 25°F (8–14°C) except for some chocolate or delicate cakes which might burn. High temperatures help to "set" the batter before the cells formed by leavening gases can expand too much. Cookies may or may not need a temperature increase.

Oven baking time — Decrease due to higher temperatures. For microwave baking, add 1–3 minutes if cake falls at end of bake time when the door is opened.

Leavening — To prevent excess rising, reduce baking powder ⅛ teaspoon at 3000 feet (0.6 ml–914 m), ⅛ – ¼ teaspoon at 5000 feet (0.6–1.25 ml–1524 m), ¼ teaspoon at 7000 feet (1.25 ml–2134 m). Reduce soda in quick breads, muffins, pancakes/waffles by ¼ of total amount.

Sugar — For each one cup (236 ml), decrease 0–1 tablespoon at 3000 feet (0–15 ml at 914 m), 2–3 tablespoons at 5000 feet (30–45 ml at 1524 m), 4–5 tablespoons at 7000 feet (60–75 ml at 2134 m). NOTE: Fast evaporation of water leads to a higher concentration of sugar, which raises the temperature when the structure sets and may cause the cake to fall. Therefore, sugar is decreased and liquid increased.

A sticky, overly browned crust and/or dip in center indicates excess sugar.

Liquid — To compensate for greater evaporation in cakes and quick breads, increase liquid. For each one cup (250 ml) add 1–2 tablespoons at 3000 feet (15–30 ml at 914 m), 2–4 tablespoons at 5000 feet (30–60 ml at 1545 m), or 3–4 tablespoons at 7000 feet (45–60 ml at 2134 m). In cookies, add ½–2 teaspoons (2.5–10 ml) water per recipe with the flour addition. If biscuit dough seems dry, add 1 tablespoon per one cup (15 ml/236.6 ml) flour.

Flour — Because flour strengthens the structure, for each recipe, add 1–4 tablespoons at 5000 feet (15–60 ml at 1545 m) and 2–5 tablespoons at 7000 feet (30–75 ml at 2134 m). Cookies squeezed through a press may need less flour. For self-rising flour, use only high altitude adjusted recipes.

Eggs — Because eggs strengthen the structure and add liquid, use large eggs, although some cooks prefer extra-large eggs. For angel food, sponge, or foam-type cakes or soufflés, it is important not to beat too much air (leavening) into the eggs. Use cold eggs, beat whites to soft peaks that just fold over; do not beat until stiff and dry. For foam-leavened cakes, using less sugar, more flour, and a higher baking temperature also helps. For a four-egg popover recipe, add 1 more egg and decrease shortening, if listed. Above 7500 feet (2286 m) an extra egg can help the structure of rich cakes.

Fats/Oils — Excess fat weakens the cell structure. For high fat-high sugar quick breads, fat may need to be reduced 2–8 tablespoons (30–120 ml) per recipe. For waffles add 1 teaspoon (5 ml) extra oil to prevent sticking.

Pans — Use larger pan size or increase number of pans. Example: For two 8-inch rounds (20 cm), use three 8-inch (20 cm) or two 9-inch (23 cm) rounds. If a large hollow air hole develops in quick breads, increase pan size or number of muffins. Generous "greasing" (1–2 tablespoons per pan—12–30 ml per pan) and flouring (if required) helps prevent sticking.

Hints: For microwaved cakes, begin with recipes developed for microwave use. Changes may not be needed, but if the cake does not rise as high, falls, has a wet center, or is too tender, then adjustments are recommended.If the center bottom is underdone, bake on an inverted plate.

Sea level recipes for cookies, bar cookies, and brownies may give acceptable, but different results at high altitudes. It is best to bake a test cookie to determine if more flour, liquid, or temperature changes are needed. NOTE: Cookies continue to brown a little after removal from oven, so cookies should be baked to a lighter color than desired. Because high altitude cookies are more delicate, cool 1 minute on baking sheet and carefully remove to rack. These changes may be needed for microwaved bar cookies or brownies, too.

For "mushroomed" muffins, adjust recipe for the altitude and increase number of muffins.

For pancakes, check that the insides are not doughy when the surfaces appear brown.

Commercial mixes — In cake, muffin, brownie, and other mixes, ingredients cannot be removed; therefore adjustments for conventional/microwave mixes are: adding flour, liquid, and/or an egg, plus increasing pan size or number of pans, or baking temperature/time. Follow the high altitude directions printed on the mix boxes, or contact the food manufacturer for information on adjustments.

Yeast breads — Rising time can be from 15 to 30 minutes shorter; let dough rise just until it doubles. Better flavor is developed by punching down the dough twice. During rising, loosely cover dough with foil or plastic wrap to prevent a dry crust from forming. Automatic bread machine recipes may require experimentation to prevent too dry a dough, or over-rising. Sometimes yeast is reduced and liquid added.

Pies, pastry, cheesecake, and soufflés — For slightly dry pastry dough, add water by ½ teaspoon until the dough cleans the bowl. Thoroughly prick unfilled crusts to prevent bubbling. (See page 17, Fruits and Steamed Puddings.) Custard and pumpkin pies may need high-sided pie plates. Baked cheesecakes may have higher sides and a center area that "settles back" during cooling. Cheesecakes require much experimentation to adjust. (For soufflés, see Eggs, page 19.)

For questions about other commercial food products, contact the food manufacturer. They may have high altitude directions on file.

MICROWAVE COOKING

BASICS

Microwave ovens designed for home use vary in size and in the features they offer. Depending on the size of the oven, the magnetron that generates microwaves may range from 600 to 800 watts for compact ovens to between 850 to 1,650 watts for midsize or large ovens. The higher the wattage, the shorter the time period needed to heat or cook a food. When microwaves penetrate food, the molecular friction generates heat; heating also occurs by conduction.

Most microwave ovens have a turntable that rotates food for uniform heating. Numeric keypads offer a number of settings for various power levels and cooking times. Many ovens also have sensors to determine when food is done and thus prevent undercooking or overcooking.

Although many ovens are equipped with temperature sensing probes, most microwave heating is controlled by adjusting the time according to the cooking power, the mass and density of the food, and its starting temperature. The glass tray on the bottom of the countertop oven elevates food to allow microwaves to reach the bottom of the food. It should not be removed during cooking. Do not operate oven without either food or liquid in it.

Cooking power may not be evenly distributed throughout the oven; however, new features are minimizing this problem. Microwave ovens designed for cooking more than one food at a time are constructed intentionally so that different amounts of energy are directed into different areas of the oven. Manufacturers are always updating their microwave ovens and products. Refer to the manufacturer's directions for use and care of the specific oven being used.

Estimating Cooking Power (wattage)
In a 4-cup (1 liter) glass measuring cup, add 2 cups (500 ml) water. Record temperature of water. Microwave on high/full power for 1 minute. Record temperature. Subtract first temperature from second temperature and multiply this by 17.5 = actual wattage. Repeat this three times and figure the average of the three. Wattage should also be listed on the manufacturer's plate on the oven.

Testing Distribution of Cooking Power
Microwaves are directed by a stirrer fan, carousel tray, or baffle, but they still may not always be directed evenly; hence, food may cook unevenly. To avoid uneven cooking, rotate dish (¼ turn) or stir food half way through cooking time.

To test distribution of power, select test material, such as cake batter. Place an equal amount of test material in 9 to 12 identical containers such as custard cups. Space containers of test material evenly throughout the oven. Turn oven on full power for 2 minutes. Greater concentration of power will be indicated by visible signs of cooking in certain areas of the test product. Water (equal amounts) also may be used for this test. The difference in water temperature from unit to unit may be determined after 2 minutes of heating. Higher water temperatures indicate a greater concentration of power in that area.

Mass and Shape of Food
As the mass of food increases, the length of time required to heat or cook increases. The relationship approaches linearity, but varies with each food. The major heating by microwaves penetrates only the outer 1-inch (2.5 cm) of the food. The center of large masses of food must be heated by conduction of heat from hot portions during a "standing" period

following heating. "Standing time" or "carry-over cooking" allows the food to rest and continue cooking. The amount of time will vary depending on the size, volume, moisture and fat content, and density of the food. Standing time averages will usually be: 1–3 minutes for individual or small items; 5 minutes for vegetables, sauces and cakes; 10 minutes for dense main dishes; and 15 minutes for large items such as roasts and turkeys. Avoid additional cooking until standing time is completed. If necessary, add cooking time in increments of 1–2 minutes to avoid overcooking.

Techniques for Promoting Even Heating

Cooking may be assisted by subdividing food into uniform or smaller portions, rotating or stirring periodically, or periodically inverting large portions of food during cooking. Foods arranged in a circle cook more uniformly than they do in a rectangle. Avoid irregular shapes and square corners, or shield edges of foods that are thin, with a postage-sized piece of foil* during cooking. Foil must not touch the side of the oven. Roasts and turkeys should be covered with foil after cooking (during standing or resting time) so the cooked meat will finish cooking and come up to finished cooking temperature. Place the thicker or denser portions of food toward the outside of the container or arrange food in a doughnut shape. Do not overcook food. Allow for standing time after cooking. Do not remove cover during standing time.

For foods requiring long cooking times, use reduced power for part of the cooking, or manually cycle the energy on and off at intervals. The "off" interval allows time for the temperature to equalize in the food.

Initial Temperature of Food

The lower the initial temperature of the food, the longer the time required to achieve the desired end temperature by heating. Starting with frozen food increases the time even more, because additional energy is required to melt the ice (latent heat of fusion). Most foods except vegetables are thawed before cooking. Thawing may be done in the microwave oven by using reduced power prior to the actual cooking period.

Density of Food

The more dense the food, the greater the amount of microwave energy required for heating. When pieces of foods differing in density or thickness are heated simultaneously, the less dense or thinner portions should be placed near the center of the container. For example, place peas in the center of a ring of mashed potatoes.

Water Content

Free water is the most polar food constituent and the most reactive to microwaves. The rapid conversion of water to steam, which occurs in microwave heating, necessitates the puncturing of food membranes or skins to prevent the food from exploding. Fats also heat very rapidly when subjected to microwaves.

When frozen foods are heated, pockets of free water can form and become superheated, resulting in an explosive release of steam. The defrost cycles on microwave ovens provide energy intermittently by pulsing on and off (cook–rest), allowing time during the off cycle for helping to equalize the temperature in the food and heating to the center of large pieces of food. Covering, during defrosting helps to distribute the heat more evenly. Food also will need to be rotated.

Reheating Foods

Reheating foods is one of the microwave oven's greatest assets. Reheat refrigerated leftovers in serving containers, allowing 3–4 minutes/pound (0.5 kg). Frozen cooked foods will need a rest-cook cycle with rotation. To reheat foods on a dinner plate, loosely cover and allow 1–2 minutes on full power. Bread products are porous and will heat fast. A roll will heat in 10–15 seconds and may still feel cool to touch. Allow carry-over time before heating again to avoid a tough, hard roll. Slotted roasting racks are helpful to reheat bread products wrapped in a paper towel or napkin. For each cup of pasta or rice, allow 1–2 minutes to reheat.

Heed your manual and warranty for the use of foil or metal in your microwave.

MICROWAVES AND FOOD SYSTEMS

Meat, Poultry, Fish

Tender, boneless cuts of meat are more suitable for microwave cooking than less tender cuts. Ground beef patties, thin steaks, or chops may be cooked with high power. For roasts, reduce cooking power, particularly after the meat is hot. Reduce power during the entire cooking period to slow the process for tenderization of pot roasts. Less tender cuts can be cooked in a microwave but may require the same amount of cooking time as required for nonmicrowave cooking to tenderize collagen sufficiently. Recommendations for promoting even heating also are applicable to cooking meats by microwaves.

Roasts may need 15–30 minutes of standing time for conduction of heat to the center of the roast after microwave cooking is stopped. From 5–15 minutes of standing time is needed for fish or poultry, depending on the size. The slower the cooking and the smaller the mass, the shorter the standing time required.

Microwaved Meat and Foods	Fahrenheit	Celsius
Beef, pork, lamb	145°	63°
Ground beef, pork, lamb	160°	71°
Poultry*	165°	74°
Fish	145°	63°
Egg dishes	160°	71°
Casseroles	160°	71°
Reheated leftovers	165°	74°

* Do not cook whole, stuffed poultry in a microwave oven; the waves might not heat the interior sufficiently to destroy harmful bacteria.

Use only thermometers designed for microwave ovens, or use a conventional thermometer when the oven is turned off. If the meat does not achieve the desired internal temperature during the standing period, it can be sliced, covered, and cooked a few minutes longer without detrimental effects to eating quality.

An even coating of fat (about 0.5 cm thick) provides a means of basting a roast during microwave cooking. Roasts or turkeys usually cook at 7 min/lb. Juices from the roast or turkey can be used to baste the meat. Halfway through cooking, place a piece of foil* on top of the meat. This will prevent the meat from being overcooked by the magnetron tube in the microwave oven. A 1" strip of foil* around the top edge of prime rib and other roasts with outer fat will stop the fat from overcooking and producing toughened meat.

Fat that collects at the bottom of the container during roasting should be removed midway during cooking so that it will not splatter.

Because less evaporation occurs than with conventional heating, only about ¼ cup (50 ml) liquid is required for moist heat cookery of less tender cuts of meat. If a pot roast is large, cut it into chunks to lessen the time required to heat the interior to a temperature sufficient to start solubilization of collagen.

Small portions of meat, poultry, or fish should be turned once during cooking. Place whole birds breast side down first and turn over midway in the cooking process. The larger the mass, the more often it should be turned. The skin of whole poultry or poultry pieces should be pierced in several places prior to cooking.

Browning aids, such as a browning tray or coatings, may be preferred for meat patties, steaks, or chops. Coatings will be less crisp than with conventional cooking. Crisping can be achieved by placing the product under a conventional broiler after cooking. For products that tend to become dry, such as pork chops, cover with sauce.

Heed your manual and warranty for the use of foil or metal in your microwave.

Milk, Cheese, and Eggs

Milk tends to foam excessively when heated to the boiling point by microwaves. Therefore, a larger container is required for heating milk alone or for casseroles and other foods containing large amounts of milk. Products containing cheese should be cooked at reduced power or for a very short time to prevent a rubbery texture. Eggs or egg-milk combinations cook fast, so the time span is reduced between optimum coagulation and over coagulation. Slow cooking and close attention are necessary. As a rule, egg foams and products composed largely of egg foam are less satisfactory when cooked by microwaves than when cooked conventionally.

Starch Pastes, Pasta, Rice

Since gelatinization of starch is enhanced by rapid heating, starch cookery is suited to microwave heating. Periodic stirring is necessary for lump free starch-thickened sauces. The sauce should be brought to a boil to achieve maximum thickening, but boiling should not be continued because the swollen starch granules may rupture. Rice and pasta require time to absorb moisture. They cook well by microwaves, but little time is saved by this method of cookery. Additional time, at reduced power, will be necessary after the water has been brought to a boil. Adding a small amount of oil reduces the tendency to boil over. Pasta, rice, or cereal may be cooked for individual servings or in quantity. Cook in a dish large enough to boil water without boiling over.

Sugar Solutions

Microwave cooking of sugar solutions minimizes the problems of scorching and of crystal build-up on the sides of the cooking container. With candy, the solution can be brought to a rapid boil, and boiling can be continued at a reduced level of microwave power. A large container is essential to prevent boiling over. Jams or preserves can be made in small batches by microwave heating. The power should be reduced after the mixture has reached the boiling point to minimize the possibility of overcooking.

Vegetables and Fruits

Vegetables and fruits are easily cooked by microwaves. The speed of cooking favors the retention of color and pleasing flavor. Overcooking may result in a rubbery texture. For vegetables that require short cooking by conventional methods, little time is saved by microwave heating. However, for long-cooking vegetables, such as whole potatoes, time may be reduced as much as 85 or 90 percent. Many vegetables can be cooked without added water, but for those with a high cellulose content, texture is improved by cooking with a small amount of water. Most vegetables and fruits should be covered. Skins on whole vegetables serve as a cover and should be pierced to permit steam to escape and to minimize the possibility of explosions. Microwave cooking brings out the natural flavoring in vegetables. Colors and flavors of vegetables are enhanced.

Baked Products

Cakes, muffins, and other quick breads cook well by microwaves but do not form brown crusts. Leavening should be reduced by one-third for microwave cooking. For products prepared from mixes, the texture may be improved by allowing the batter to stand for 15–20 minutes before cooking. The surface of the products will appear slightly moist when cooking is complete. Allow 10–12 minutes standing time for layer cakes so that some cooking will continue for a short time. Lining the container with waxed paper will reduce the tendency for sogginess on the bottom of the cake. Biscuits, yeast bread, cookies (other than bar cookies), and cakes without shortening are less satisfactory when cooked by microwaves than when baked conventionally.

Fats and Oils

Fats and oils heat rapidly when exposed to microwaves. However, they do not heat uniformly, which can result in very dangerous spattering of hot fat and uneven cooking. Therefore, deep fat frying in a microwave is not recommended.

Baby Food

Because microwaves heat unevenly, avoid using the microwave oven to thaw or heat breast milk, formula, or baby-food meat, meat sticks, eggs, or foods with high fat content which can cause overheating. Excess heat also can destroy nutrient quality. Baby foods with low fat content can best be heated in a dish (not a jar) at 15-second increments, stirred, and held to stand for 30 seconds. Testing of foods should be done before feeding to make sure the food is not too hot.

PREPARATION OF MEALS BY MICROWAVES

Heat long-cooking foods and those that hold heat well first. Allow for continued cooking (particularly in large masses of food) after the microwave heating has stopped. If more than one food is cooked at one time, extend the length of time. Cooking time must be adjusted according to the amount of food cooked at one time. Use a microwave oven for partial cooking of some foods. Take advantage of this appliance for fast defrosting and for fast reheating of foods. Plan meals for the characteristics of microwave heating, such as less evaporation of liquid, greater expansion of leavened products, rapid evolution of steam, and continued heating after oven is turned off, particularly in dense foods. Remember that casseroles and entrees will require only about one-fourth to one-third as long for microwave as for conventional cooking. An interruption for testing doneness will not be detrimental to the finished quality of any product.

Adapting Conventional Recipes

Use successful microwave recipes as a guide to modify conventional recipes. Consider the major ingredients and their suitability for microwave cooking. Use small recipes first, as they are easier to convert than large recipes. Recipes with a large amount of moisture may need adjusting, as the microwave does not evaporate as much liquid. A general rule is to reduce the liquid in the conventional recipe by one-fourth. To determine cooking time, consider that 1 cup (250 ml) of tap water boils and 1 cup of food heats in 1½ to 3 minutes on high. If the oven takes longer, add additional time to recipes. To be more accurate, weigh food and estimate 6–7 minutes/pound (0.5 kg) on high, depending on oven wattage. Increase cooking time as the amount of food increases. Other considerations are shape, volume, weight, density, initial temperature, oven wattage, peak electric use hours, and the cooking container. Undercook when experimenting with new foods and recipes and then continue to cook if more time is judged to be needed.

High Altitude

Adjust conventional recipes by increasing flour ¼ cup (60 ml) and liquid by ⅓ cup (80 ml). Boiling occurs at a lower temperature, so it may take longer (1–2 minutes) to cook dense foods.

Choosing Utensils

Choose utensils that are microwave safe (glass, paper, china without metal rim). Some equipment, plastic containers, plastic wraps, and films are designated as microwave safe. Take-out containers, plastic margarine, or whipped topping containers can warp, melt, or contain harmful chemicals (Bisphenol A[BPA], polycarbonate plastics, etc.).

Test dishes for microwave use by placing one cup (250 ml) of tap water and an empty dish in oven. Heat on high for one minute. If the water gets hot and the dish does not, it can be used. Use only glass-ceramic dishes if oven has infrared browner. Metal reflects microwaves; if recommended by manufacturer, foil may be used for shielding. Use only thermometers designed for microwave ovens. However, conventional thermometers can be used to test the temperature of food when the oven is turned off.

As covers, use casserole lids, plastic film, paper plates, waxed paper, paper towels, or napkins. Covering food traps heat and speeds up the cooking time. Choose porous materials, such as paper towels, if the surface of the food is dry. If possible, use round containers for cooking instead of those with square corners. A heatproof glass may be used in the center of casseroles to achieve the doughnut shape. Special microwave browning dishes are heated empty in the microwave to absorb energy. The bottom of the dish absorbs energy instead of transmitting it, thus causing the food to brown when placed on the very hot surface.

Reducing the Speed of Cooking

To retard the rate of cooking, utilize oven controls for reducing power, cycle energy on and off manually, or introduce an additional load, such as a container of water to absorb part of the energy.

Safety

Home canning is not recommended because there is no way of knowing how much pressure is building inside the sealed jar. Home canned vegetables and meats should be processed conventionally to ensure destruction of all *Clostridium botulism* spores. Cooking sponge cakes, deep-fried foods, popovers, hard and soft-cooked eggs in the shell are not recommended. Follow manufacturer's recommendations for cooking popcorn. Do not operate a microwave oven empty. If the cavity does not have enough food mass, the microwaves may bounce back to the magnetron tube and shorten the life of the oven. Cooking containers will become hot to the level of food in the container as heat in the food transfers to the container. Use hot pads as a precaution. Transfer frozen, prepackaged convenience and frozen prepared food to nonmetal containers for cooking. To clean a microwave oven, heat 1 cup (250 ml) water until it steams. Wipe inside of cavity with soft cloth after steam softens food. Microwave ovens are always being updated, hence the need to follow manufacturer's direction for use and care of oven. To remove food odors, add lemon juice or baking soda to warm water, close oven door and let mixture sit for a short time.

Enhancing Appearance of Food

The speed of microwave cooking and the tendency for food to give up heat to the surrounding atmosphere are not conducive to browning and crusting of the surfaces of food. Browning occurs if the food requires cooking for 20 minutes or more. Many foods are acceptable without a brown crust. Browning ingredients and sauces may be used to advantage on other foods.

TO ENHANCE FOOD APPEARANCE

Biscuits	Brown using browning tray. Top with toasted sesame seeds, poppy seeds, cinnamon and sugar, or dry onion mix.
Cakes	Sprinkle brown sugar and cinnamon in container before pouring batter, or sprinkle on top after cooking. Use topping for upside-down cakes. Cool baked cake and then ice it.
Casseroles	Top with toasted bread crumbs, crushed chips, cereals, toasted nuts, canned onion rings, chopped bacon, or brown under broiler before or after cooking by microwave.
Fish	Top or coat with toasted crumbs or nuts. Cover with sauce. Glaze with brown sugar or other ingredients. Brown on grill or broil and complete cooking by microwave. Use browning utensil.
Meat, Poultry	Brush with brown sauce or gravy mix. Sprinkle with paprika or dry onion soup.
Pastry	Prepare with milk instead of water. Add a few drops of food coloring. When making quiche, brush uncooked crust with Worcestershire sauce, then micro-cook for 2 minutes.

SLOW-COOKER COOKING

The slow cooker is an electrical appliance, specifically designed to cook foods slowly, generally taking 4 to 12 hours. There are at least two general types of slow cookers. One has a stoneware or crockery container in an electrical heating base. Heating elements often wrap around the sides of the stoneware and control settings may include low and high. Another type of slow cooker consists of a metal container that is heated from the bottom. The temperature control may include a variety of temperature settings, but a range for slow-cooking will be specifically noted. Variations of these two types, such as a crockery bowl in a metal cooking pot with an adjustable thermostat, are also available. Check the manufacturer's instructions for information on using a specific slow cooker, and note the recommended cooking times and settings. Always cook for the suggested time on the proper setting. The slow cooker is helpful in cooking less tender cuts of meat, soups, and stews. A variety of other dishes, including casseroles, vegetables, beans, hot drinks and cereals can also be prepared in a slow cooker. For cooks who wish to adapt favorite recipes to the slow cooker, this information provides a guide.

Adapting Recipes
- Look for steps that may be omitted (for example, browning aspects). Most ingredients can be added at the beginning of the cooking period.

- For most recipes, one cup of liquid is sufficient, but a general rule of thumb is to use only one-half as much as in a standard recipe. Additional amounts may be needed if cooking a product such as pasta or rice, which absorbs liquid.

- Crushed or ground seasonings should be added near the end of cooking because they become too mild during the long cooking period. Whole seasonings may withstand the long cooking, and their flavor may intensify, so use about one-half as much as usual.

- Rice and pasta become gummy with long cooking; add them during the last hour of cooking. If pasta is to be cooked before adding to the slow cooker, cook the pasta just until al dente.

- Sour cream and milk curdle during long cooking and should be added during the last 30 minutes. Condensed soups are satisfactory for the longer cooking times and may be substituted for milk or cream.

Food Placement
Placement of foods in the cooker may determine the success or failure of the dish. Vegetables such as potatoes, carrots, and onions cook very slowly and should be kept small to medium in size and placed in the bottom of the pot. This also allows the meat juices to drip over the vegetables, enhancing their flavor. Unless the meat is very fatty, a rack usually is not necessary. If a sauce is used over meat or vegetables, it should be poured evenly over the food.

Timing Factors
- Allow plenty of cooking time, especially on low. Remember that timing is generally not critical and an extra hour will not greatly affect the food. Always cook the food until it is completely done and tender.

- The temperature of the food when placed in the cooker will affect the cooking time. Most cooking times are based on using refrigerated foods. Frozen foods require a longer cooking time than refrigerated foods. In some slow cookers, frozen foods are not recommended or specific instructions must be followed; check the use and care manual for information on frozen foods in a specific slow cooker.

- The volume of food will affect the cooking time. Refer to the use and care manual as a guide for the amount of food suited to the size of cooker being used. Generally the cooking times are based on units one-half to three-fourths full. Do not overfill slow cookers. If cooking a very small amount of food in a cooker with a wrap-around heating element, the cooking time may be shortened, and the cooking progress should be checked.

- If there is much fat present, meat should first be trimmed, browned, or broiled to eliminate as much fat as possible.

- Minerals (as in some hard water areas) and acids increase the cooking time in dried legumes and may affect other foods in hard-water areas. Sugars and acid foods such as tomatoes and molasses should be added only after the legumes have been softened completely.

- Some foods should be added during the last 1 to 2 hours of cooking including seafood, canned or frozen vegetables, and fresh mushrooms. Frozen vegetables and seafood should be thawed before being added to the cooker.

The following chart provides guidelines for cooking adapted recipes in a slow cooker.

TIME GUIDE FOR SLOW COOKER*

If Recipe Says:	Time in Slow Cooker	
	High Setting	Low Setting
15 to 30 min.	1.5 to 2.5 hrs.	4 to 6 hrs.
35 to 45 min.	3 to 4 hrs.	6 to 10 hrs.
50 min. to 3 hrs.	4 to 6 hrs.	8 to 18 hrs.

* Courtesy of Rival Manufacturing Company

CONVECTION OVEN COOKING

A convection oven uses forced hot air to speed the baking/roasting process, thus saving time in the oven.

Types of Ovens
Convection ovens are available as countertop, wall, or range ovens. The three different convection modes are: convection with heating element located around the fan and outside the oven cavity; convection bake with heating elements on inside oven cavity and a fan to circulate the hot air; and microwave/convection—a combination of microwave power and heating element and fan located outside the oven cavity. Factors to consider when adapting conventional recipes to the convection oven include time, temperature settings, and type of bakeware. Check the appliance manual for specific suggestions.

Baking
Temperature — Oven temperature is decreased by 25–50°F (15–30°C). Bakes items with sufficiently brown surface but undercooked centers may need the temperature lowered an additional 25°F (15°C) and increased baking time.

Time — Baking time varies with moisture content, richness, and depth of product. Check times in appliance manual. Generally for convection or convection bake modes, times can be reduced as follows: thin items—about 1–2 minutes; cakes—5 minutes; and large turkeys—up to 30 percent. Preheating is necessary only for food baked less than 20 minutes and products such as popovers where steam rising is important.

Size — Large items may not cook fully in the center. Divide these into small units such as two or three loaves instead of one.

Roasting
Temperature — Use the same temperature as conventional recipes. Preheating is not necessary. Roast meats uncovered, except turkey, which should be covered once it is golden brown.

Time — Reduce the time by one-third depending on the size of product. If meat is too rare in the center, lower the temperature and increase the time.

Controlling Moisture — Baste roasts with glaze or barbecue sauce only during the last 10 to 20 minutes; use a drip pan with ¼ inch (0.8 cm) water. Frozen meat can be roasted in the same time as thawed meat in a conventional oven.

Quantity Cooking

A major benefit of convection ovens is quantity cooking. It is possible to bake three racks of cookies, biscuits, pizzas, or similar items at the same time and have even browning of the product.

Bakeware

Metal bakeware such as aluminum and heavy-duty aluminum foil gives the greatest time savings, followed by cast iron and black steel. Ceramic and glass dishes require conventional baking time. Baking sheets should have only one edge. Shallow pans that allow at least 1 to 1½ inches (2.5–3.7 cm) of space between the bakeware and the oven wall are recommended for roasting. Covered casseroles can be used in the convection oven, but the convection benefit of reduced time is minimized. Cookware should be centered in front of the fan with 1 inch (2.5 cm) air space on all sides.

FOOD LABELING

Federal laws governing food labeling are the concern of the following agencies:

FDA — Food and Drug Administration. A federal agency empowered to enforce five specific laws relating to checking all foods and food additives for safety, purity, and wholesomeness (Federal Food, Drug and Cosmetic Act; Fair Packaging and Labeling Act; Radiation Control and Health Safety Act; Public Health Service Act; and Nutrition Labeling and Education Act of 1990). FDA officers inspect plants where food is processed. The agency is also responsible for the accuracy and correctness of information of packages and labels on the majority of foods.

USDA — U.S. Department of Agriculture. This department is responsible for meat and poultry safety, quality, and labeling (see FSIS). The Research Service of this agency conducts food and nutrition research. Areas investigated include effects of processing and cooking on nutrient content of food and food preferences and habits of individuals and groups. Officers inspect plants for the cleanliness of the plant and workers and health of the animals slaughtered.

FSIS — Food Safety and Inspection Service. This agency of USDA inspects all red meats and poultry for purity, wholesomeness, and truthful labeling. This agency monitors meat and poultry for hazardous residues above Environmental Protection Agency (EPA) levels.

AMS — Agricultural Marketing Service. This agency within USDA grades fresh, frozen, canned and dehydrated vegetables into levels of quality. It also establishes grade standards for most fresh and processed fruits and for fresh meat, poultry, and eggs.

USDC NMFS — U.S. Department of Commerce–National Marine Fisheries Service. This agency provides voluntary inspection of fish and fish products. The service develops standards and specifications for quality, conditions, quantity, grade and packaging of fish, processing plants, and fish products.

USPHS — U.S. Public Health Service. This agency safeguards the purity of dairy products. Evidence of contamination is monitored according to standards stated in the Grade A Pasteurized Milk Ordinance. This agency assists with enforcement of standards relating to sanitation, taste, odor, and milkfat content. The federal code defines milk fat standards for various milk products. This agency works with USDA in monitoring processing at milk plants.

Ingredient Labeling

For nonmeat and nondairy products, the ingredient label is regulated by FDA. Meat and dairy product labels are regulated by USDA. The ingredient label must tell the name of a product, the form it is in, and identify anything this has been added to it. Ingredients must be listed by weight, from highest weight to lowest content. The Nutrition Labeling and Education Act of 1990 established requirements for the declaration of all ingredients in standardized foods, declaration of certified color additives in foods, declaration of sources of protein hydrolysates, and declaration on the nutrition label of percentage of a fruit or vegetable juice in a beverage claiming to contain such a juice.

The effective date for total percentage juice labeling, and ingredient labeling of standardized foods and certified colors was May 8, 1993.

Organic Foods

Many foods on the market today have been produced by organic farming methods. This means they have been grown without the use of chemical fertilizers, insecticides, or chemical herbicides. Instead organic farmers use sustainable farming methods, apply natural fertilizers such as manure or compost, use natural means of controlling insect pests, rotate crops, till, and mulch to control weeds.

The USDA has established the following standards for labeling of organic foods sold to consumers:

100% organic – Products that are completely organic or made of all organic ingredients.

Organic – Products that are at least 95% organic.

Made with organic ingredients – Products that contain at least 70% organic ingredients.

Only products that are at least 95% organic can carry the USDA Organic seal on the package.

Nutrition Labeling

The Nutrition Labeling and Education Act (NLEA) of 1990 brought about a great many changes to the labeling practices monitored by the FDA. Proposed rules for implementing the act were reviewed throughout 1992, with final rules published in the Federal Register on January 6, 1993. The effective date for mandatory nutrition labeling using the specified format was May 8, 1994.

The purpose of the labels is to allow comparison of foods for nutritional content. The 1990 law requires mandatory nutritional labeling of most foods offered for sale and regulated by FDA. The nutrition label is required to include information on total calories and calories from fat and on amounts of total fat, saturated fat, cholesterol, sodium, total carbohydrates, dietary fiber, sugars, protein, vitamin A, vitamin C, calcium and iron—in that order. Manufacturers also may voluntarily declare information on calories from saturated fat and on amounts of polyunsaturated and monounsaturated fat, soluble and insoluble fiber, sugar, alcohol, other carbohydrate, potassium, additional vitamins and minerals for which Reference Daily Intakes (RDIs) have been established, and the percent of vitamin A present as beta-carotene. The information presented on the label is to represent the packaged product prior to consumer preparation.

The standard format for nutrition information on food labels consists of:

1. The quantitative amount per serving of each nutrient except vitamins and minerals

2. The amount of each listed nutrient as a percent of the Daily Value for a 2,000 kilocalorie diet

3. A footnote with reference values for selected nutrients based on 2,000 kilocalorie and 2,500 kilocalorie diets

4. Kilocaloric conversion information

Voluntary labeling applies to fresh produce and seafood unpackaged or packaged at retail. Nutrition information at point of purchase may be presented via large placards, brochures, or videos. Unless claims are made about the following nutrients, labeling is voluntary: kilocalories from saturated and unsaturated fat, total carbohydrates, protein; unsaturated fat or amounts of polyunsaturated and monounsaturated fats (g); insoluble and soluble fiber; protein as percentage of RDI for foods other than infant foods; potassium (mg), thiamin, riboflavin, niacin, and other vitamins and minerals as percentage of RDI unless added as a supplement. Nutrition information is given "as consumed" for raw fish and "as packaged" for raw fruits and vegetables. Sixty percent of retailers surveyed must be in compliance for at least 90 percent of the 20 most frequently consumed raw fruits, raw vegetables, and raw fish.

The USDA-Food Safety and Inspection Service (FSIS) also published in the January 6, 1993 issue of the

Federal Register final rules amending the federal meat and poultry products inspection regulations permitting voluntary nutrition labeling on single-ingredient, raw meat and poultry products, and mandatory nutrition labeling for all other meat and poultry products. The FSIS rules were an effort to parallel as much as possible the nutrition labeling regulations of the NLEA. The effective date for USDA nutrition labeling of meat and poultry products was July 6, 1994.

Nutrition Profile

The Food and Drug Administration (FDA) regulations established Reference Daily Intakes (RDIs) and Daily Reference Values (DRVs). The final rules published in 1993 retained the values established by FDA in 1973 for vitamins and minerals but changed the terms for those values from U.S. Recommended Daily Allowances (U.S.RDA) to Reference Daily Intake (RDI). The regulation also established label reference values for eight other nutrients, including fat, cholesterol, and fiber. The values were established as Daily Reference Values (DRVs). To avoid confusion, all reference values on food labels are referred to as Daily Values, or DVs.

Reference Serving Sizes

Serving sizes are defined as the amount of food customarily consumed per eating occasion. Nutrient content values listed on product labels are then based on the standardized serving sizes. A total of 184 food product categories have been defined—139 by FDA, 23 for meats by FSIS, and 22 for poultry by FSIS. Additionally, there are specific rules for single-serving containers and items that come in discrete units such as slices of bread or individual muffins or cookies.

Descriptive Terms

FDA has defined the terms "free," "low," "light" or "lite," "reduced," "less," and "high," as well as "good source," "very low" (for sodium only), "lean," "extra lean," "fewer," "more," and "added" (for "fortified" or "enriched").

Some of the specific definitions are as follows: Criteria for the term "low" are based on reference serving sizes or for products having reference amounts of less than 30 g or 2 tablespoons, per 50 g, and thus low fat is a food with not more than 3 g of fat, low calorie is a food with not more than 40 calories, and low sodium is a food with not more than 140 mg sodium.

Light (lite) can be used if the food has one-third fewer kilocalories than a comparable product, if half of the kilocalories are from fat and the fat has been reduced by 50 percent; and cholesterol-free claims may be made only on foods that contain 2 g or less of saturated fat per reference serving.

The terms "high" and "good source" are based on a percentage of the DV of the specific nutrients in a reference serving. "High" is defined as 20 percent or more of the DV, and "good source" as between 10 and 19 percent of the DV. See Table 1.4 for a more complete list of nutrient content labeling claims definitions.

Health Claims

FDA allows food manufacturers to make unqualified health claims on food labels based on "significant scientific agreement" or an "authoritative statement of a scientific body of the U.S. government or the National Academy of Sciences." (See www.fda.gov/aboutfda/centersoffices/officeoffoofs/cfsan/default.htm for more information.) FDA also permits other qualified health claims when there is emerging evidence of a relationship between a food or dietary supplement and reduced risk of a disease or health-related condition, structure and function claims, and statements of dietary guidance that are truthful and non-misleading. Health claims link various nutrients (i.e., dietary fat, sodium, and calcium) and food groups (i.e., fruits and vegetables and fiber-containing grain products) to reduction in risk of diseases such as coronary heart disease, cancer, hypertension, osteoporosis, and other diseases. Structure/function claims that describe the role of a nutrient or dietary ingredient in affecting structure or function in the human body also are allowed by FDA. Some examples of various types of claims are in Table 1.4.

TABLE 1.4
EXAMPLES OF HEALTH CLAIMS FOR NUTRITION LABELS

Type of Claim	Example Food	Food	Model Claim
Unqualified	Sodium and hypertension	Low sodium	Diets low in sodium may reduce risk of high blood pressure, a disease associated with many factors.
Unqualified	Dietary fat and cancer	Low fat	Development of cancer depends on many factors. A diet low in total fat may reduce the risk of some cancers.
Qualified	Walnuts and heart disease	Whole or chopped walnuts	Supportive but not conclusive research shows that eating 1.5 ounces per day of walnuts, as part of a low saturated fat and low cholesterol diet and not resulting in increased caloric intake, may reduce the risk of coronary heart disease.
Structure/Function	Calcium	Dairy foods	Calcium builds strong bones.

Trans Fat Content

Beginning January 2006, food manufacturers were required by FDA to list trans fat content of foods in grams separately on the Nutrition Facts label in two circumstances:

1. The food contains over 0.5 g trans fat per serving

2. A health claim is made about fat, fatty acids, or cholesterol

The requirement to include trans fat on the label is based on emerging scientific evidence linking consumption of trans fats to increased risk of coronary heart disease. FDA has not yet established a Daily Value for trans fats. Consumers are advised to use the food label information as a guide for choosing foods low in saturated fat, trans fat, and cholesterol.

Food Allergens

The Allergen Labeling and Consumer Protection Act, which became effective in January 2006, is designed to provide specific information to consumers regarding major food allergens contained in foods. Foods with any ingredient containing egg, wheat, peanuts, milk, tree nuts, soy, fish, or crustaceans (shellfish) are required to state the common name of the food in parentheses or an additional statement in the ingredient list on the product label.

Nutrient Content Claims and Standardized Foods

The large number of substitute products now in the marketplace has created a need for standardization of the substitutes. The substitute product cannot be nutritionally inferior to the original product. The substitute product also must have similar performance characteristics to the original product, and if it does not, this must be clearly printed on the label. The product must contain the ingredients used in the original product, but also may contain certain safe and suitable ingredients, provided the product is not nutritionally and functionally inferior to the original food in its performance characteristics.

TABLE 1.5

NUTRIENT CONTENT LABELING CLAIMS DEFINITIONS

Definition by Food Energy/Nutrient Category							
Descriptive Term	Calories	Fat	Saturated Fat	Cholesterol	Sodium	Sugars	Comments
Free	Contains no amount of, or only trivial amounts, of any one or more of the categories: calories, fat, saturated fat, cholesterol, sodium, and sugars.						Synonyms: "no," "without," "zero"
	<5 kcal / Serving	<0.5 g/ serving	<0.5 g/ serving	<2 mg/ serving	<5 mg/ serving	<0.5 g/ serving	
Low	40 kcal or less/ serving	3 g or less/ serving	1 g or less/ serving	20 mg or less/ serving	140 mg or less/ serving	Not defined	Synonyms: "little," ("few" for calories). Amount applies/50 g food if references amount 30 g or less (small serving)
Very low					35 mg or less/ serving		
Lean		<10 g/ serving	<4 g/ serving	<95 mg/ serving			Amounts apply per 100 g also
Extra lean		<5 g/ serving	<2 g/ serving	<95 mg/ serving			Amounts apply per 100 g also
Light or lite	Contains ⅓ fewer calories than ref. food	Contains ½ fat of ref. food			Content reduced by 50% in low-calorie/low-fat food		If food gets 50% or more of calories from fat, must have 50% reduction in fat
Reduced	Nutritionally altered product has at least 25 percent less of nutrient or calories than reference product. Claim can't be made if reference food meets requirements for "low" claim.						Synonyms: "lower" ("fewer" for calories)
Less	Food, altered or not, has 25 percent less of a nutrient or calories per reference serving.						Synonym: "fewer"
High	Contains 20 percent or more of DV for nutrient per reference serving.						
More	Food, altered or not, has 10 percent or more of DV of nutrient per reference serving.						
Good source	10-19 percent of DV of a particular nutrient per reference serving.						
Fresh	May only be used on a food that is raw, never frozen or heated, and contains no preservatives.						

Exemptions from Mandatory Programs

Foods exempt from mandatory nutrition labeling requirements include:

1. Foods offered for sale by small businesses

2. Food sold in restaurants or other establishments in which food is served for immediate human consumption

3. Foods similar to restaurant foods that are ready to eat but are not for immediate consumption, are primarily prepared on site, and are not offered for sale outside of that location

4. Foods that contain insignificant amounts of all nutrients subject to the law such as coffee and tea

5. Dietary supplements, except those in conventional food form

6. Infant formula

7. Medical foods

8. Custom-processed fish or game meats

9. Foods shipped in bulk form

10. Donated foods

Otherwise exempted foods that make a nutrient content claim or health claim forfeit the exemption.

FOOD ADDITIVES

By the broadest definition, a food additive is any substance that becomes a part of the food product when added directly or indirectly.

The 1906 Food and Drug Act and the more comprehensive Food, Drug and Cosmetic Act of 1938 gave the government authority to remove adulterated and obviously poisonous foods from the market. The 1958 Food Additives Amendment, The Delaney Clause, and the 1960 Color Additives Amendment are laws specifically set up to regulate additives in foods. In these laws, legislation shifted the burden from the government to the manufacturer to prove that a food additive is safe. FDA was authorized to regulate additives only on the basis of safety. The agency has no power to limit the number of additives approved, or to judge whether an additive is really needed.

Under the Food Additives Amendment, however, two major categories of additives were exempted initially from the testing and approval process. The first group of some 700 substances belongs to the "generally recognized as safe" (GRAS) list, which includes salt and other common ingredients such as sugar and many herbs and spices, considered safe based on either a history of safe use before the Food Additives Amendment was passed in 1958 or the results of scientific studies. The GRAS list was designed to allow continued use of substances considered harmless because of past extensive use without known harmful effects. However, GRAS additives have been undergoing systematic testing for safety since 1971. Also exempted from testing were the "prior sanctioned substances," those that had been approved before 1958 for use in food by either FDA or USDA.

An additive is intentionally incorporated into foods for one or more of these four purposes:

• To maintain or improve nutritional value

• To maintain freshness

• To help in processing or preparation

• To make food more appealing

Some people have adverse reactions to certain foods and some food additives. When that happens, reactions can range from headaches or hives to seizures or death. If an allergic reaction to an additive is suspected, contact a physician for diagnosis and treatment.

Guide to Types of Additives

Nutrients	Enrich (replace vitamins and minerals lost in processing) or fortify (add nutrients that may be lacking in the diet).	**Maturing and Bleaching Agents, Dough Conditioners**	Accelerate the flour aging process; improve baking qualities of flour.
Preservatives (Antimicrobials)	Prevent food spoilage from bacteria, molds, fungi and yeast; extend shelflife; or protect natural color or flavor.	**Anticaking Agents**	Prevent caking, lumping, or clustering of a finely powdered or crystalline substance.
Antioxidants	Delay / prevent rancidity or enzymatic browning.	**Flavor Enhancers**	Supplement, magnify, or modify the original taste and / or aroma of food without imparting a characteristic flavor of their own.
Emulsifiers	Help to distribute evenly tiny particles of one liquid into another; improve homogeneity, consistency, stability, or texture.	**Flavors**	Heighten natural flavor; restore flavors lost in processing.
Stabilizers, Thickeners, Texturizers	Impart body; improve consistency or texture; stabilize emulsions; affect mouth feel.	**Colors**	Give desired, appetizing, or characteristic color of food.
Leavening Agents	Affect cooking results – texture and volume.	**Sweeteners**	Make the taste of food more agreeable or pleasurable.
pH Control Agents	Change / maintain acidity or alkalinity.	**Alternative Sweeteners**	Make the taste of food sweeter with no or few added calories.
Humectants	Cause moisture retention.	**Fat Substitutes**	Affect the mouth feel of foods by replacing fat with fat substitutes.

Additives

Key to abbreviations used in following list:

Stabil-thick-tex	=	stabilizers-thickeners-texturizers
Leavening	=	leavening agents
pH control	=	pH control agents
Mat-bleach-condit	=	maturing and bleaching agents, dough conditioners
Anticaking	=	anticaking agents

Acetic acid (vinegar)..................................... pH control

Acetone Peroxide ....mat-bleach-condit

Acesulfame-K. ....sweetener

Agar.. stabil-thick-tex

Alginate .... stabil-thick-tex

Aluminum, sodium sulfate .... pH control
    firming agent

Ammonium alginate..................................... pH control

Annatto extract ....color

Arabingalactan (larch gum)................... stabil-thick-tex

Ascorbic acid (Vitamin C)............ nutrient, antioxidant

Aspartame..sweetener

Beet powder ....color

Benzoyl peroxide.............................. mat-bleach-condit

Benzoic acid ....preservative (sodium benzoate)

Beta-carotene.. nutrient, color

BHA (butylated hydroxyanisole)................ antioxidant

BHT (butylated hydroxytoluene) .... antioxidant

Calcium bromate...............................mat-bleach-condit

Calcium carbonate .... anticaking

Calcium caseinate...... stabil-thick-tex nutrient (fortify)

Calcium phosphate .... leavening
    (monocalcium phosphate) pH control nutrient

Calcium propionate ....preservative

Carob bean gum .... stabil-thick-tex

Caramel...color

Carrageenan.. stabil-thick-tex

Carrot oil...color

Cellulose .... stabil-thick-tex

Chlorine and chlorine dioxide ....mat-bleach-condit

Citric acid .... pH control, antioxidant

Cyclamate...sweetener
   (legal in Canada, illegal in U.S.)

Diglycerides ....emulsifier

DSG (disodium 5'-guanylate)..............flavor enhancer

EDTA.......antioxidant (ethylene-diaminetetra-acetate)

Ethyl vanillin.. flavor

Ferrous gluconate.................................... nutrient, color

Ferrous sulfate (iron) .... nutrient

FD and C Colors ....color
   Blue 1
   Blue 2
   Green 3
   Orange B
   Citrus Red
   Citrus Red 2
   Red 3 (provisional)
   Red 40
   Yellow 5
   Yellow 6

Gelatin.. stabil-thick-tex

Glutamic acid.. flavor

Glycerine ....humectant

Grape skin extract ....color

Guar gum .... stabil-thick-tex

Gum arabic (acacia) .... stabil-thick-tex

Heptyl paraben..preservative

Hydrogen peroxide.......................... mat-bleach-condit

HVP....................................... flavor enhancer
(hydrolyzed vegetable protein)
Iron-ammonium citrate .... anticaking
Iron, reduced... nutrient
Isopropyl citrate .... antioxidant
Lactic acid.................................pH control preservative
Lecithin .... emulsifer
Limonene..antioxidant, flavor
Locust bean gum. .... stabil-thick-tex (carob bean)
Magnesium silicate .... anticaking
Mannitol. ....sweetener
Methyl cellulose ... anticaking, stabil-thick-tex bulking
Methyl paraben ....preservative
Modified food starch .... stabil-thick-tex
Monoammonium glutamate.................flavor enhancer
Monoglyceride...emulsifier
Monosodium Glutamate (MSG) ....flavor enhancer
Niacinamide.. nutrient
Nitrates ....preservative
Oleoresins.. flavor
Parabens ....preservative
Pectin... stabil-thick-tex
Phosphoric acid .... pH control
Polysorbates (60, 65, 80) .... emulsifiers
Potassium bromate ....mat-bleach-condit
Potassium iodide (iodine)................................. nutrient
Proprionic acid & salts ....preservative
Propylene glycol..................................... stabil-thick-tex
Propyl gallate..................................... antioxidant
Riboflavin .... nutrient, color
Saccharin ....sweetener

Saffron..color
Silicon dioxide .... anticaking
Simplesse®..fat substitute
Sodium ascorbate (Vitamin C) .... nutrient
Sodium citrate... pH control
Sodium erythorbate .... antioxidant
Sodium proprionate....................................preservative
Sodium stearyl fumarate...................mat-bleach-condit
Sorbic acid ....preservative
Sorbitan monostearate......................................emulsifier
Sorbitol....................................flavoring, humectant
Stearyl lactylate ....emulsifier, conditioner,
whipping agent
Sugar (fructose, invert sugar, glucose,
sucrose, dextrose).. sweeteners
Sulfite salts ....preservative
Sulfur dioxide ....preservative
Tartaric acid (cream of tartar)...................... pH control
TBHQ ....antioxidant (tertiary butyl hydro-quinone)
Thiamin.. nutrient
Titanium dioxide...color
Tocopherols (Vitamin E)...............nutrient, antioxidant
Tragacanth gum...................................... stabil-thick-tex
Trisodium phosphate.......................... stabil-thick-tex
Turmeric ....color
Vanilla .... flavor
Vanillin.. flavor
Vitamin A.. nutrient

SUPPLEMENTARY AIDS TO FOOD PREPARATION

BAKING TEMPERATURES AND TIMES
OVEN TEMPERATURES

Type of Product	°F	°C	Baking Time (minutes)
Breads			
Biscuits	425–450	220–230	10–15
Corn bread	400–425	200–220	30–40
Cream puffs	425–450	220–230	45–60
Muffins	400–425	200–220	20–25
Popovers	350–375	180–190	
Quick loaf breads	350–375	180–190	60–75
Yeast bread	400	200	30–40
Yeast rolls, plain	400–425	200–220	15–25
sweet	375	190	20–30
Cakes with fat			
Bundt	350	180	40–45
Cupcake, 12 cups	350–375	180–190	15–25
Layer, 9 inch	350–375	180–190	20–25
Loaf	350	180	45–60
Cakes without fat			
Angel food and sponge	350–375	180–190	30–45
Jelly roll	325	160	22–28
Cookies			
Drop	350–400	180–190	8–15
Rolled	375	190	8–15
Meringues	200	(100)	60 + 120 after oven off

BAKING TEMPERATURES AND TIMES (CONTINUED)
OVEN TEMPERATURES

Type of Product	°F	°C	Baking Time (minutes)
Egg, meat, milk, and cheese dishes			
Cheese soufflé, custards (baked in a pan of hot water)	350	180	45–60
Macaroni and cheese	350	180	25–30
Meat loaf	350	150	60–90
Rice pudding (raw rice)	300	150	120–180
Scalloped potatoes	350	180	60–75
Pastry			
One-crust pie (custard type), unbaked shell	400–425	200–220	30–40
Meringue on warm cooked filling in prebaked shell	350	180	12–15
Shell only	450	230	10–12
Two crust pies with uncooked filling	400–425	200–220	45–55
Two crust pies with cooked filling	425–450	220–230	30–45

NOTE: When baking in ovenproof glassware, reduce oven temperature by 25°F or by 10°C.

NOTE: For packaged mixes, follow directions on package.

SOLUBILITY OF SALT (SODIUM CHLORIDE)
AMOUNT OF SALT TO SATURATE 100 G WATER

Temperature	Grams	%
-4°F (-20°C)	30.9	23.6
68°F (20°C)	36.0	26.4
212°F (100°C)	39.8	28.2

SUBSTITUTION OF INGREDIENTS

For	Substitute
1 Tbsp flour (15 ml) (used as thickener)	1½ tsp (7 ml) cornstarch, potato starch, rice starch, or arrowroot starch; 1 Tbsp (15 ml) quick cooking tapioca
1 c (250 ml) sifted all-purpose flour	1 c (250 ml) unsifted all-purpose flour minus 2 Tbsp (30 ml), if spooned into cup
1 c (250 ml) sifted cake flour	⅞ c (225 ml) sifted all-purpose flour, or 1 c minus 2 Tbsp (225 ml) sifted all-purpose flour
1 c (250 ml) sifted self-rising flour	1 c (250 ml) sifted all-purpose flour plus 1½ tsp (7 ml) baking powder and ½ tsp (2 ml) salt
1 c (250 ml) dark corn syrup	¾ c (175 ml) light corn syrup and ¼ c (50 ml) light molasses
1 c (250 ml) corn syrup	1 c (250 ml) sugar plus ¼ c (50 ml) liquid*
1 c (250 ml) light brown sugar	½ c (125 ml) dark brown sugar plus ½ c (125 ml) granulated sugar
1 c (250 ml) honey	1¼ c (300 ml) sugar plus ¼ c (50 ml) liquid*
1 ounce (28 g) semisweet chocolate	½ ounce (14 g) unsweetened baking chocolate plus 1 Tbsp (15 ml) sugar
1 ounce (28 g) unsweetened chocolate	3 Tbsp (50 ml) cocoa plus 1 Tbsp (15 ml) fat
1 c (250 ml) coffee cream (20% fat)	3 Tbsp (50 ml) butter plus about ⅞ c (255 ml) milk
1 c (250 ml) heavy cream (40% fat)	⅓ c (75 ml) butter plus about ¾ c (175 ml) milk
1c (250 ml) whole milk	1 c (250 ml) reconstituted nonfat dry milk plus 2½ tsp (12 ml) butter or margarine, or ½ c (125 ml) evaporated milk plus ½ c (125 ml) water
1 c (250 ml) milk	3 Tbsp (50 ml) sifted regular nonfat dry milk plus 1 c (250 ml) water, or ⅓ c (75 ml) instant nonfat dry milk plus 1 c (250 ml) minus 1 Tbsp water
1 c (250 ml) buttermilk or sour milk	1 Tbsp (15 ml) vinegar or lemon juice plus enough sweet milk to make 1 c (250 ml), let stand 5 minutes, or 1¾ tsp (8 ml) cream of tartar plus 1 c (250 ml) sweet milk
1 c (250 ml) sour cream	1 c (250 ml) plain yogurt or ⅞ c (225 ml) sour milk plus ⅓ c (75 ml) butter
1 c (250 ml) buttermilk	1 c (250 ml) plain yogurt
1 c (250 ml) milk	1 c (250 ml) buttermilk and omit 1 tsp (5 ml) baking powder, replacing with ½ tsp (2 ml) soda and 1 tsp (5 ml) shortening
1 c (250 ml) butter	⅞ c (225 ml) oil

SUBSTITUTION OF INGREDIENTS (CONTINUED)

For	Substitute
1 tsp (5 ml) baking powder	¼ tsp (1 ml) baking soda plus ⅝ tsp (3 ml) cream of tartar; or ¼ tsp (1 ml) baking soda plus ½ cup (125 ml) fully soured milk or buttermilk; or ¼ tsp (1 ml) baking soda plus ½ Tbsp (7 ml) vinegar or lemon juice used with sweet milk to make ½ c (125 ml); or ¼ tsp (1 ml) baking soda plus ¼ to ½ c (50 ml to 125 ml) molasses; or ¼ tsp (1 ml) baking soda plus ½ c (125 ml) yogurt
2¼ tsp (11.25 ml) active dry yeast	1 package active dry yeast, or 1 compressed yeast cake
1 whole egg	2 egg yolks, or 3 Tbsp (50 ml) plus 1 tsp thawed frozen egg, or 2 Tbsp (30 ml) and 2 tsp dry whole egg powder plus an equal amount of water
1 egg yolk	3½ tsp (17 ml) thawed frozen egg yolk, or 2 tsp (10 ml) dry egg yolk plus 2 tsp (10 ml) water
1 egg white	2 Tbsp (30 ml) thawed frozen egg white, or 2 tsp (10 ml) dry egg white plus 2 Tbsp (30 ml) water
1 c (250 ml) bread crumbs	¾ c (175 ml) cracker crumbs
1 c (250 ml) tomato juice	½ c (125 ml) tomato sauce plus ½ c (125 ml) water
1 medium clove garlic	⅛ tsp (0.5 ml) garlic powder or ¾ tsp (3 ml) garlic salt
1 tsp (5 ml) lemon juice	½ tsp (2 ml) vinegar
1 tsp (5 ml) grated lemon peel	¼ to ½ tsp (2 ml) lemon extract
1 small onion	1 tsp (5 ml) onion powder or 1 tsp (5 ml) minced dry onion

* Use whatever liquid is called for in the recipe.

NOTE: The amounts of corn syrup and honey are based on the way these products function in recipes and not on the sweetness equivalence with sugar.

TABLE 1.6

TEMPERATURE CONVERSION TABLE

The numbers in the body of the table give in degrees F the temperature indicated in "Degrees C" at the top and side. To convert 178°C to Fahrenheit scale, find 17 in the column headed "Degrees C." Proceed in a horizontal line to the column headed 8, which shows 352°F as corresponding to 178°C. To convert 352°F to Celsius scale, find 352 in the Fahrenheit readings, then in the column headed "Degrees C," find the number which is on the same horizontal line, i.e., 17. Next, fill in the last number from the heading of the column in which 352 was found, i.e., 8, resulting in 178°C, which is equivalent to 352°F.

Range	Conversion Formulae
-29°C (-20°F) to 309°C (588°F)	$T°C = 5/9\ (T°F-32)$
	$T°F = 9/5\ (T°C+32)$

TEMPERATURE CONVERSION TABLE (CONTINUED)

Degrees °C	0	1	2	3	4	5	6	7	8	9
-2	-4°F	6°F	8°F	-9°F	-11°F	-13°F	-15°F	-17°F	-18°F	-20°F
-1	14°F	12°F	10°F	9°F	7°F	5°F	3°F	1°F	0°F	2°F
-0	32°F	30°F	28°F	27°F	25°F	23°F	21°F	19°F	18°F	16°F
0	32°F	34°F	36°F	37°F	39°F	41°F	43°F	45°F	46°F	48°F
1	50°F	52°F	54°F	55°F	57°F	59°F	61°F	63°F	64°F	66°F
2	68°F	70°F	72°F	73°F	75°F	77°F	79°F	81°F	82°F	84°F
3	86°F	88°F	90°F	91°F	93°F	95°F	97°F	99°F	100°F	102°F
4	104°F	106°F	108°F	109°F	111°F	113°F	115°F	117°F	118°F	120°F
5	122°F	124°F	126°F	127°F	129°F	131°F	133°F	135°F	136°F	138°F
6	140°F	142°F	144°F	145°F	147°F	149°F	151°F	153°F	154°F	156°F
7	158°F	160°F	162°F	163°F	165°F	167°F	169°F	171°F	172°F	174°F
8	176°F	178°F	180°F	181°F	183°F	185°F	187°F	189°F	190°F	192°F
9	194°F	196°F	198°F	199°F	201°F	203°F	205°F	207°F	208°F	210°F
10	212°F	214°F	216°F	217°F	219°F	221°F	223°F	225°F	226°F	228°F
11	230°F	232°F	234°F	235°F	237°F	239°F	241°F	243°F	244°F	246°F
12	248°F	250°F	252°F	253°F	255°F	257°F	259°F	261°F	262°F	264°F
13	266°F	268°F	270°F	271°F	273°F	275°F	277°F	279°F	280°F	282°F
14	284°F	286°F	288°F	289°F	291°F	293°F	295°F	297°F	298°F	300°F
15	302°F	304°F	306°F	307°F	309°F	311°F	313°F	315°F	316°F	318°F
16	320°F	322°F	324°F	325°F	327°F	329°F	331°F	333°F	334°F	336°F
17	338°F	340°F	342°F	343°F	345°F	347°F	349°F	351°F	352°F	354°F
18	356°F	358°F	360°F	361°F	363°F	365°F	367°F	369°F	370°F	372°F
19	374°F	376°F	378°F	379°F	381°F	383°F	385°F	387°F	388°F	390°F
20	392°F	394°F	396°F	397°F	399°F	401°F	403°F	405°F	406°F	408°F
21	410°F	412°F	414°F	415°F	417°F	419°F	421°F	423°F	424°F	426°F
22	428°F	430°F	432°F	433°F	435°F	437°F	439°F	441°F	442°F	444°F
23	446°F	448°F	450°F	451°F	453°F	455°F	457°F	459°F	460°F	462°F
24	464°F	466°F	468°F	469°F	471°F	473°F	475°F	477°F	478°F	480°F
25	482°F	484°F	486°F	487°F	489°F	491°F	493°F	495°F	496°F	498°F
26	500°F	502°F	504°F	505°F	507°F	509°F	511°F	513°F	514°F	516°F
27	518°F	520°F	522°F	523°F	525°F	527°F	529°F	531°F	532°F	534°F
28	536°F	538°F	540°F	541°F	543°F	545°F	547°F	549°F	550°F	552°F
29	554°F	556°F	558°F	559°F	561°F	563°F	565°F	567°F	568°F	570°F
30	572°F	574°F	576°F	577°F	579°F	581°F	583°F	585°F	586°F	588°F

TABLE 1.7

BASIC RECIPE PROPORTIONS

The following table shows proportions of ingredients to one another in certain basic recipes. The amounts of ingredients do not constitute full-size recipes and are not intended for family meal preparation. Weights are given for situations where ingredients are being weighed. Metric conversions can be done on the basis of 1 cup equals 236.6 milliliters and 1 teaspoon equals 5 milliliters.

Product	Flour[1]	Liquid	Fat	Eggs	Sugar	Salt	Baking Powder[2]	Other Ingredients
BEVERAGES								
Cocoa and Chocolate		1 c milk 242 g			2 tsp–1 Tbsp 8.3–12.5 g	few grains		1 Tbsp cocoa 7 g or ½ oz chocolate 14.2 g
Coffee		¾ c water 178 g						1 Tbsp coffee 5.3 g
Instant		¾ c water 178 g						1–2 tsp instant coffee 0.8–1.6 g
Freeze Dried		¾ c water 178 g						⅓ tsp 0.5 g
Tea		¾ c water 178 g						½–1 tsp tea 0.75–1.5 g
BREADS								
Biscuits	1 c 115 g	⅓–½ c milk 12.6–47.2 g	2–4 Tbsp 23.6–47.2 g			½ tsp 3 g	1¼–2 tsp 4.5 or 5.8 g	
Griddle Cakes (pancakes)	1 c 115 g	¾–⅞ c milk 181.5–211.8 g	1 Tbsp 11.8 g	½ 25 g	0–1 Tbsp 0–12.5 g	½ tsp 3 g	1½ or 2 tsp 5.4 or 5.8 g	
Muffins	1 c 115 g	½ c milk 121 g	2–3 Tbsp 23.6–35.4 g	½ 25 g	1–2 Tbsp 12.5–25 g	½ tsp 3 g	1¼ or 2 tsp 4.5 or 5.8 g	

BASIC RECIPE PROPORTIONS (CONTINUED)

Product	Flour[1]	Liquid	Fat	Eggs	Sugar	Salt	Baking Powder [2]	Other Ingredients
BREADS								
Popovers	1 c 115 g	1 c milk 242 g	1–2 Tbsp 11.8–23.6 g			¼–¾ tsp 1.5–4.5 g		
Waffles	1 c 115 g	¾–1 c milk 181.5–242 g	1–3 Tbsp 11.8–35.4 g	1–2 50–100 g		½ tsp 3 g	1¼ or 2 tsp 4.5 or 5.8 g	
Yeast Bread	1 c 115 g	⅓ c milk 80.7 g	0–1 Tbsp 0–11.8 g		1 tsp– 1 Tbsp 4.2–12.5 g	¼ tsp 1.5 g		¼ compressed yeast cake 12.8 g or ¼ small package active dry yeast 1.7 g
CAKES AND PASTRY								
Cake with fat	1 c cake or all-purpose 96 or 115 g	¼–½ c milk 60.5–121 g	2–4 Tbsp 23.6–47.2 g	½–1 25–50 g	½–¾ c 100–150 g	⅛–⅓ tsp 0.75–1.5 g	1 or 2 tsp 3.6–5.8 g	flavoring
Chiffon	1 c cake 96 g	⅓ c water 79 g	¼ c (salad oil) 52.5 g	1 150 g	⅔ c 134 g	½ tsp 3 g	1¼ or 1½ tsp 4.5–5.4 g	¼ tsp cream of tartar 0.8 g flavoring
Cake without added fat								
Angel Food	1 c cake 96 g			1–1½ c whites 246–369 g	1¼–1½ c 250–300 g	½ tsp 3 g		¾–1½ tsp cream of tartar 2.3–4.6 g flavoring
Sponge	1 c cake 96 g	0–3 Tbsp water 0–44.4 g		5–6 250–300 g	1 c 200 g	½ tsp 3 g		0–¾ tsp cream of tartar 0–2.3 g flavoring
Cream Puffs	1 c 115 g	1 c water 237 g	½ c 144	4 200 g		¼ tsp 1.5 g		
Doughnuts	1 c 115 g	¼ c milk 60.5 g	1 tsp 3.9 g	½ 25 g	¼ c 50 g	¼ tsp 1.5 g	1 or 2 tsp 3.6–5.8 g	flavoring
Pastry	1 c 115 g	2–3 Tbsp water 29.6 g	4–5½ Tbsp 47.2–58.8 g			½ tsp 3 g		

BASIC RECIPE PROPORTIONS (CONTINUED)

Product	Flour[1]	Liquid	Fat	Eggs	Sugar	Salt	Baking Powder[2]	Other Ingredients
EGG DISHES								
Custards		1 c milk 242 g		1–1⅔ 50–83.5 g	1½–3 Tbsp 18.8–37.5 g	⅛ tsp 0.75 g		flavoring
Omelets		1 Tbsp 151.1 g		1 50 g		⅛ tsp 0.75 g		seasonings
Soufflés Entrée	¼–⅓ c ¾ Tbsp 21.6—28.8 g	1 c milk 242 g	3–4 Tbsp 35.2—47.2 g	3 150		¼–½ tsp 1.5–3 g		seasonings
PUDDINGS								
Cornstarch		1 c milk 242 g		0–1 0–50 g	2–3 Tbsp 25–37.5 g	⅛ tsp 0.75 g		1–1½ Tbsp cornstarch 8–12 g flavoring
Gelatin, Jellies Plain		2 c milk, water fruit juices or other liquid 484 g			2 Tbsp 25 g			1 envelope gelatin 1 Tbsp 7–10 g
Fruit or vegetable		3 c liquid 741 g			¼ c 50 g	few grains		2 envelopes gelatin 2 Tbsp 14–20 g
Bavarian Creams		2 c milk 484 g		4 200 g	¼ c 50 g			2 envelopes gelatin 2 Tbsp 14–20 g 2 c fruit pulp 484 g 1 c whipping cream 242 g flavoring

BASIC RECIPE PROPORTIONS (CONTINUED)

Product	Flour[1]	Liquid	Fat	Eggs	Sugar	Salt	Baking Powder[2]	Other Ingredients
PUDDINGS								
Tapioca		1 c milk 242 g		½–1 25–50	2 Tbsp 25 g	⅛ tsp 0.75 g		1½ Tbsp quick cooking tapioca 14.25 g flavoring
Rice (steamed)		1 c milk 242 g			1–2 Tbsp 12.5–25 g	⅛ tsp 0.75 g		2–4 Tbsp raw rice 22.8– 45.5 g flavoring
Rice (baked)		1 c milk 242 g	1 Tbsp 11.8 g		1 Tbsp 12.5 g	few grains		1 Tbsp raw rice 11.4 g flavoring
SAUCES								
White wine sauce								
Thin	1 Tbsp 7.8 g	1 c milk 242 g	1 Tbsp 11.8 g			¼ tsp 1.5 g		pepper, if desired
Medium	2 Tbsp 15.6 g	1 c milk 242 g	2 Tbsp 23.6 g			¼ tsp 1.5 g		pepper, if desired
Thick	3–4 Tbsp 23.4– 31.2 g	1 c milk 242 g	3–4 Tbsp 35.4– 47.2 g			¼ tsp 1.5 g		pepper, if desired
Fruit sauce		1 c fruit juice 247 g			1–4 Tbsp 25–50 g			¼–1 Tbsp cornstarch 6–8 g fruit, if desired
SOUPS								
Cream with nonstarchy vegetables	1 Tbsp 7.8 g	1 c milk 242 g	1 Tbsp 11.8 g			¼ tsp 1.5 g		seasonings, vegetables
Cream with starch vegetables	1½ tsp 3.7 g	1 c milk 242 g	1 Tbsp 11.8 g			¼ tsp 1.5 g		seasonings, vegetables

[1] All-purpose flour unless cake flour is specified.

[2] Use the smaller amount with SAS-phosphate powder and the larger amount with quick acting powder.

TABLE 1.8
CONVERSION TO METRIC UNITS

Comparison of Avoirdupois and Metric Units of Weight									
1 oz	=	0.06 lb	=	28.35 g	=	(30 g)*	1g	=	0.035 oz
2 oz	=	0.12 lb	=	56.70 g	=		2g	=	0.07 oz
3 oz	=	0.19 lb	=	85.05 g	=		3g	=	0.11 oz
4 oz	=	0.25 lb	=	113.40 g	=	(125 g)	4g	=	0.14 oz
5 oz	=	0.31 lb	=	141.75 g	=		5g	=	0.18 oz
6 oz	=	0.38 lb	=	170.10 g	=		6g	=	0.21 oz
7 oz	=	0.44 lb	=	198.45 g	=		7g	=	0.25 oz
8 oz	=	0.50 lb	=	226.80 g	=	(250 g)	8g	=	0.28 oz
9 oz	=	0.56 lb	=	255.15 g	=		9g	=	0.32 oz
10 oz	=	0.62 lb	=	283.50 g	=		10g	=	0.35 oz
11 oz	=	0.69 lb	=	311.85 g	=		11g	=	0.39 oz
12 oz	=	0.75 lb	=	340.20 g	=	(350 g)	12g	=	0.42 oz
13 oz	=	0.81 lb	=	368.55 g	=		13g	=	0.46 oz
14 oz	=	0.88 lb	=	369.90 g	=		14g	=	0.49 oz
15 oz	=	0.94 lb	=	425.25 g	=		15g	=	0.53 oz
16 oz	=	1.00 lb	=	453.59 g	=	(500 g)	16g	=	0.56 oz

*Figures in parentheses indicate common use.

CONVERSION TO METRIC UNITS (CONTINUED)

Comparison of U.S. and Metric Units of Liquid Measure

1 fl oz	=	29.573 ml	1 qt	=	0.946 l	1 gal	=	3.785 l
2 fl oz	=	59.15 ml	2 qt	=	1.89 l	2 gal	=	7.57 l
3 fl oz	=	88.72 ml	3 qt	=	2.84 l	3 gal	=	11.36 l
4 fl oz	=	118.30 ml	4 qt	=	3.79 l	4 gal	=	15.14 l
5 fl oz	=	147.87 ml	5 qt	=	4.73 l	5 gal	=	18.93 l
6 fl oz	=	177.44 ml	6 qt	=	5.68 l	6 gal	=	22.71 l
7 fl oz	=	207.02 ml	7 qt	=	6.62 l	7 gal	=	26.50 l
8 fl oz	=	236.59 ml	8 qt	=	7.57 l	8 gal	=	30.28 l
9 fl oz	=	266.16 ml	9 qt	=	8.52 l	9 gal	=	34.07 l
10 fl oz	=	295.73 ml	10 qt	=	9.46 l	10 gal	=	37.85 l

Comparison of U.S. and Metric Units of Liquid Measure

1 ml	=	0.034 fl oz	1 l	=	1.056 qt	1 l	=	0.264 gal
2 ml	=	0.07 fl oz	2 l	=	2.11 qt	2 l	=	0.53 gal
3 ml	=	0.10 fl oz	3 l	=	3.17 qt	3 l	=	0.79 gal
4 ml	=	0.14 fl oz	4 l	=	4.23 qt	4 l	=	1.06 gal
5 ml	=	0.17 fl oz	5 l	=	5.28 qt	5 l	=	1.32 gal
6 ml	=	0.20 fl oz	6 l	=	6.34 qt	6 l	=	1.59 gal
7 ml	=	0.24 fl oz	7 l	=	7.40 qt	7 l	=	1.85 gal
8 ml	=	0.27 fl oz	8 l	=	8.45 qt	8 l	=	2.11 gal
9 ml	=	0.30 fl oz	9 l	=	9.51 qt	9 l	=	2.38 gal
10 ml	=	0.34 fl oz	10 l	=	10.57 qt	10 l	=	2.64 gal

TABLE 1.9

HYDROGEN ION CONCENTRATION AND PH OF SOME COMMON FOODS

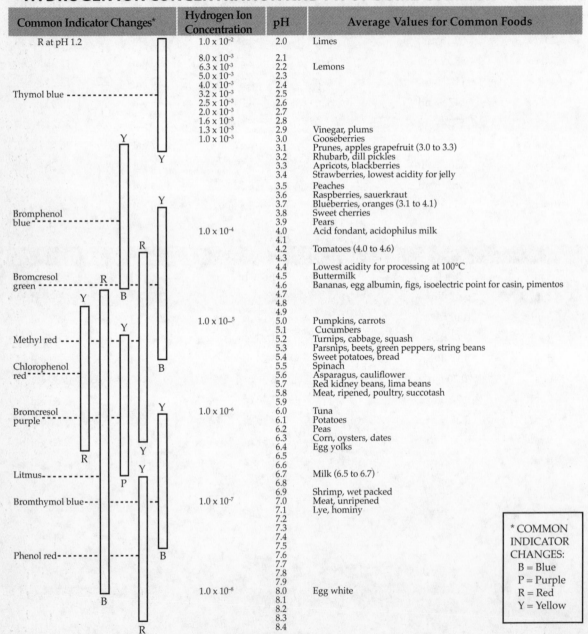

Common Indicator Changes*	Hydrogen Ion Concentration	pH	Average Values for Common Foods
R at pH 1.2	1.0×10^{-2}	2.0	Limes
	8.0×10^{-3}	2.1	
	6.3×10^{-3}	2.2	Lemons
	5.0×10^{-3}	2.3	
	4.0×10^{-3}	2.4	
Thymol blue	3.2×10^{-3}	2.5	
	2.5×10^{-3}	2.6	
	2.0×10^{-3}	2.7	
	1.6×10^{-3}	2.8	
	1.3×10^{-3}	2.9	Vinegar, plums
	1.0×10^{-3}	3.0	Gooseberries
		3.1	Prunes, apples grapefruit (3.0 to 3.3)
		3.2	Rhubarb, dill pickles
		3.3	Apricots, blackberries
		3.4	Strawberries, lowest acidity for jelly
		3.5	Peaches
		3.6	Raspberries, sauerkraut
		3.7	Blueberries, oranges (3.1 to 4.1)
Bromphenol blue		3.8	Sweet cherries
		3.9	Pears
	1.0×10^{-4}	4.0	Acid fondant, acidophilus milk
		4.1	
		4.2	Tomatoes (4.0 to 4.6)
		4.3	
		4.4	Lowest acidity for processing at 100°C
Bromcresol green		4.5	Buttermilk
		4.6	Bananas, egg albumin, figs, isoelectric point for casin, pimentos
		4.7	
		4.8	
		4.9	
	1.0×10^{-5}	5.0	Pumpkins, carrots
		5.1	Cucumbers
Methyl red		5.2	Turnips, cabbage, squash
		5.3	Parsnips, beets, green peppers, string beans
		5.4	Sweet potatoes, bread
Chlorophenol red		5.5	Spinach
		5.6	Asparagus, cauliflower
		5.7	Red kidney beans, lima beans
		5.8	Meat, ripened, poultry, succotash
		5.9	
Bromcresol purple	1.0×10^{-6}	6.0	Tuna
		6.1	Potatoes
		6.2	Peas
		6.3	Corn, oysters, dates
		6.4	Egg yolks
		6.5	
		6.6	
Litmus		6.7	Milk (6.5 to 6.7)
		6.8	
Bromthymol blue		6.9	Shrimp, wet packed
	1.0×10^{-7}	7.0	Meat, unripened
		7.1	Lye, hominy
		7.2	
		7.3	
		7.4	
		7.5	
Phenol red		7.6	
		7.7	
		7.8	
		7.9	
	1.0×10^{-8}	8.0	Egg white
		8.1	
		8.2	
		8.3	
		8.4	

* COMMON INDICATOR CHANGES:

B = Blue
P = Purple
R = Red
Y = Yellow

TABLE 1.10

TEMPERATURE OF FOOD FOR CONTROL OF BACTERIA

°C	°F	
121	250	116°C to 121°C – Canning temperature for low-acid vegetables, meat, fish, and poultry in pressure canner
116	240	
		102°C to 106°C – Jam/Jelly stage
100	212	**Boiling Point**
85		100°C – Temperature of boiling water at sea level; temperature to can fruits, jams, jellies, preserves, low-acid tomatoes, and pickles in a water-bath canner
		85°C to 100°C – Simmering
		80°C – Scalding
80	180	Cooking temperatures destroy most bacteria. The time required to kill bacteria is less as temperature increases.
		60°C to 83°C – Pasteurizing
74	165	End cooking temperature for eggs, meat, poultry, and seafood varying with product, cut, and desired doneness
60	140	Warming temperatures prevent bacterial growth, but allow the survival of some bacteria.
57	135*	Some bacterial growth may occur at this temperature; many bacteria survive.
	125	**DANGER ZONE: Temperatures in this zone allow rapid growth of bacteria and production of toxins by some bacteria.** (Do not keep foods in this temperature zone for more than 2–3 hours.)
35	95	
	60	35°C – Lukewarm
		26°C to 32°C – yeast dough rises
		15°C to 60°C – rennin, an enzyme, is active
10	50	4°C to 60°C – These temperatures allow the growth of bacteria and mold that cause
5	41	foodborne illness.
	40	≤ 5°C (≤ 41°F) Optimum refrigerator storage: Temperature for thawing frozen foods
2	36	(Cold temperatures permit slow growth of some bacteria that cause spoilage.)
0	32	**Freezing Point**
		Freezing temperatures stop growth of bacteria, but may not kill them.
-32	0	-32°C to -43°C – Optimum freezer storage, may vary with type of food
-43	-20	

Adapted from ServSafe Coursebook, 6th ed., National Restaurant Association Educational Foundation, 2012.

* **The USDA considers 40–140°F (4–60°C) to be the temperature danger zone for consumers. The FDA Food Code for retailers designates the zone to be 41–135°F (5–57°C).**
Amy Brown, *Understanding Food: Principles & Preparation*, 4th ed. Wadsworth/Cengage Learning: 2011, p. 81.

TABLE 1.11

THICKENING AND GELLING AGENTS

Thickening Agent	Uses and Quantity Required	Precautions in Mixing	Effect of Temperature	Other Factors that Affect Thickening	Characteristics of the Gel
Agar	**Salad and dessert jellies:** 4 to 6 g (about 2 tsp) per pt of liquid (500 ml).	Soak in 3 to 6 times the weight of cold liquid, then dissolve by bringing to a boil.	Gel forms on cooling to 104 to 113°F (40 to 45°C); softens at 176 to 185°F (80 to 85°C).	Gel strength not easily destroyed by heat or acid.	Gel rigid, short, crumbly; transparent; may have weedy odor if sample not highly purified.
Egg	**Custard puddings and sauces:** 2 to 3 medium eggs per pt (500 ml) of milk or 4 to 6 yolks.	Blend well with sugar and milk. Coagulate by slow heating.	Overcooking causes syneresis (weeping) and curdling.	Sugar and dilution raise coagulation temperature; acid lowers it. Use of water instead of milk results in a flocculent precipitate rather than a gel.	Baked custard forms firm, continuous clot. Stirred custard is soft, thickened but not set.
Flour	**Thin soup or sauce:** 2 Tbsp (16 g) per pt (500 ml) of liquid. **Medium sauces:** 4 to 5 Tbsp (32 to 40 g) per pt (500 ml) of liquid. **Soufflés, molded pastes:** ½ c per pt of liquid (125 ml/500 ml).	Disperse in cold liquid or in fat or mix with sugar before adding hot liquid. Stir while cooking.	Heat to 194°F (90°C) or above to obtain maximum thickening. Viscosity increases on cooling.	Heating with acid causes thinning. High sugar concentrations retard gelatinization and reduce thickening power.	Opaque paste.

THICKENING AND GELLING AGENTS (CONTINUED)

Thickening Agent	Uses and Quantity Required	Precautions in Mixing	Effect of Temperature	Other Factors that Affect Thickening	Characteristics of the Gel
Waxy rice flour (mochiko, sweet rice flour)	**Frozen sauces and gravies:** to prevent curdling and liquid separation 4 to 5 Tbsp per pt (32 to 40 g/500 ml) liquid. Also prevents gelation of thickening canned products.	Same as flour, but waxy rice is less likely to lump.	Maximum thickening at 158 to 176°F (70 to 80°C); little difference between hot and cold viscosity.	Heating with acid and homogenization causes thinning.	Does not gel. Forms short opaque paste.
Gelatin	**Molded desserts and salads:** 7 to 12 g (about 1 Tbsp or 1 envelope) per pt (500 ml) of liquid according to grade.	Soak in 2 to 6 times the weight in cold liquid, then dissolve by heating to 104°F (40°C) or by adding hot liquid, and then add sugar.	Gel forms after a few hours of chilling. Softens at 80°F (26.5°C) and higher.	Heating with acid causes reduction of gel strength. Raw pineapple, kiwi, and figs prevent setting because of enzyme action.	Gel firm but springy and quivery; transparent in appearance.
Gum tragacanth	**Salad dressings, sauces:** 2 to 3 g per pt (500 ml) of liquid gives thin paste; 6 to 8 g per pt (500 ml) gives thick gel.	Dissolve either in hot or cold water (dissolves much more rapidly in hot).	Little change in viscosity over a wide temperature range.	Acid, alkali or salt plus heat causes thinning.	Gel thick and mucilaginous but not rigid even at high concentrations.
Irish moss	**Puddings, sauces:** 4 to 6 g per pt (500 ml) liquid give a thick paste; 15 to 25 g per pt (500 ml) of liquid give a stiff gel.	Soak in cold water, then heat to 140°F (60°C) or above to dissolve.	Gel melts at 81 to 106°F (27 to 41°C) depending on concentration.	Acid plus heat causes thinning. Heat alone has no effect.	Gel thick and mucilaginous; becomes rigid only at high concentrations; may have weedy odor if not highly purified.
Cornstarch and rice starch	1 Tbsp cornstarch or rice starch = 2 Tbsp flour.	Same as flour.	Same as flour.	Same as flour.	Paste more translucent than flour paste.

THICKENING AND GELLING AGENTS (CONTINUED)

Thickening Agent	Uses and Quantity Required	Precautions in Mixing	Effect of Temperature	Other Factors that Affect Thickening	Characteristics of the Gel
Potato starch and arrowroot starch	1 Tbsp potato or arrowroot starch = 2 Tbsp flour (See Effect of Temperature column). Suitable for starch-egg mixtures or fruit sauces where higher temperatures are not desired.	Same as flour.	Reached maximum thickening at 158 to 176°F (70 to 80°C); higher temperature or further heating causes very marked thinning.	Same as flour, thinning also brought about by excessive stirring.	Paste very transparent.
Waxy cereal starches	Prevent gelatin and syneresis of canned products during storage—may be used in combination with flour.	Same as flour.	Similar to waxy rice flour.	Thinned by heating with acid.	Waxy starches give somewhat ropy translucent pastes.
Tapioca, pearl	About twice as much as quick-cooking tapioca.	Soak several hours before cooking.	Cook until tapioca is transparent.	Same as quick-cooking tapioca.	Same as quick-cooking tapioca.
Tapioca, quick-cooking	**Puddings:** 3 Tbsp per pt (500 ml) of liquid. **Fruit pie fillings:** 1½ to 3 Tbsp for 8- or 9-inch pie. **Soup:** 1½ to 3 Tbsp per qt (100 ml) of liquid.	Mix in cold or hot liquid; no soaking necessary.	Bring only to a boil. Mixture thickens as tapioca particles swell and become transparent. It continues to thicken while cooling.	Stir while cooking. Over-stirring while cooling tends to disrupt tapioca particles, resulting in a sticky, gelatinous mixture.	Pastes transparent, nonhomogenous (particles remain distinct). Mixture thickens as it cools. Especially satisfactory for fruit pie fillings.

FOODBORNE ILLNESSES

Foodborne disease is estimated to cause many illnesses, hospitalizations, and even deaths annually in the U. S. Illnesses occur from improper food handling practices in consumer homes and foodservice establishments, both commercial and institutional. Some population groups such as immune-compromised individuals, older adults, infants and children, and pregnant women are considered to be more highly susceptible to foodborne illness than other individuals.

The majority of cases of foodborne illness are caused by bacteria and viruses. Parasites and fungi are less common causes. Bacterial foodborne illnesses can be classified as foodborne infections, foodborne intoxications, or foodborne toxin-mediated infections.

The Bad Bug Book on the CFSAN section of the FDA website lists specific information about a variety of foodborne pathogens.

Foodborne infections occur when humans consume a food or beverage containing significant numbers of bacterial cells, and the bacteria then reproduces inside the human body. Most foodborne infections result in symptoms of abdominal pain, headache, fever, nausea, and diarrhea. Incubation periods vary according to the type of bacteria involved, and duration can range from 1 day to a week. Some of the most common bacteria causing foodborne infections and the foods in which they occur are shown below.

TABLE 1.12

EXAMPLES OF BACTERIA CAUSING FOODBORNE INFECTIONS AND ASSOCIATED FOODS

Campylobacter jejuni	Raw chicken, raw milk, and untreated drinking water.
E. Coli O157:H7	Raw and undercooked beef, alfalfa sprouts, unpasteurized fruit juice, dry-cured salami, lettuce, game meta, cheese curds, and raw milk.
Listeria monocytogenes	Raw milk, soft cheeses, ice cream, raw vegetables, fermented raw-meat sausages, raw and cooked poultry, raw meats, and raw and smoked fish.
Salmonella	Raw meats, poultry, eggs, milk and dairy products, fish, shrimp, frog legs, meat, coconut, sauces and salad dressings, cake mixes, cream-filled desserts, dried gelatin, peanut butter, cocoa, and chocolate.
Vibrio vulnificus	Oysters, clams, and crab.

Foodborne intoxications are caused when food is improperly handled, and bacteria present in the food grow and produce toxins. When humans ingest the food containing the toxin, they become ill, usually within 6 to 24 hours. Foodborne intoxications often cause symptoms of nausea, vomiting, and diarrhea, but not fever. In some cases, such as with *Clostridium botulinum*, death may result. Some of the most common bacteria causing foodborne intoxications are shown below.

TABLE 1.13

EXAMPLES OF BACTERIA CAUSING FOODBORNE INTOXICATIONS AND ASSOCIATED FOODS

Bacillus cereus	Meats, milk, vegetables, fish, rice, starchy foods (potato, pasta, and cheese products), sauces, puddings, soups, casseroles, pastries, and salads.
Clostridium botulinum	Improperly processed, canned low-acid foods (vegetables, fish, poultry, and meat).
Staphylococcus aureus	Meat and meat products, poultry and egg products, salads (protein, potato, and pasta), cream-filled pastries and cream pies, sandwich fillings, and milk and dairy products.

Foodborne toxin-mediated infections are caused when bacteria are ingested with food, but once inside the human body grow and produce a toxin that causes illness. *Clostridium perfringens*, which is found in meat, meat products, and gravy, produces this kind of illness. *Bacillus cereus* and *E. Coli O157:H7*, which cause foodborne infections, also can cause foodborne toxin-mediated infections. In children, *E. Coli O157:H7* can cause hemolytic uremic syndrome and death.

Viruses carried in food are also a common cause of foodborne illness. Unlike bacteria, viruses can only reproduce in living cells; they do not reproduce in food. Viruses are usually spread to food because of the poor personal hygiene of a food handler who is ill. They may contaminate any type of food, not just those foods that are considered potentially hazardous. Foods commonly implicated in viral foodborne illness include raw and ready-to-eat foods that are not cooked prior to consumption such as salads, raw fruits and vegetables, and sandwiches. Water and ice also can be carriers for viruses that cause illness. Viruses that commonly cause short-term illness (1 to 3 days) are *Norwalk* and *Norwalk-like virus* and *Rotavirus*. Another virus, *Hepatitis A*, can cause longer term illness ranging from 1 to 2 weeks or several months.

FDA Food Code
The *FDA Food Code*, a comprehensive guide on food safety and sanitation standards and food handling practices, is often used as the basis for state and local regulations and ordinances intended to promote public food safety. The *Food Code* is published every five years with periodic updates during the interim periods. The preface of the *Food Code* states that five major causes of foodborne illness in foodservice establishments are improper holding temperatures, inadequate cooking, contaminated equipment, food from unsafe sources, and poor personal hygiene of food handlers. Some key provisions of the food code that apply to managers and staff of foodservice operations are as follows:

- The person in charge of a food establishment must demonstrate knowledge of prevention of foodborne disease, preparation and storage of potentially hazardous foods, cleaning/sanitizing procedures, critical control points, major food allergens, and understanding of the *Food Code*.

- Employers must screen employees for illness from common food pathogens (*E. Coli, Salmonella, Hepatitis A, Shigella, and Norovirus*) and exclude or restrict those who are ill.

- Employees must wash hands with a 20-second handwashing at appropriate times.

- Employees must not touch ready-to-eat food with bare hands (except raw fruits and vegetables while washing). Foods should be handled with suitable utensils such as deli tissue, spatula, tongs, single-use gloves, or dispensing equipment.

Some key provisions of the *Food Code* that apply to foods, food handling, and food storage are:

- Potentially hazardous foods (foods needing time/temperature control) include raw or heat-treated animal foods (i.e., meat, poultry, seafood, eggs, dairy) and heat-treated plant foods. Raw seed sprouts, cut melons, cut tomatoes, cut leafy greens, garlic-in-oil mixtures, and other foods with specific combinations of high Aw (> 0.88) and low acidity (pH > 4.2) may also be considered potentially hazardous.

- Only pasteurized fruit juices and eggs should be served to highly susceptible populations.

- Shell eggs are to be stored and transported at temperatures no greater than 45°F.

- Three acceptable ways of thawing frozen foods are: place in a refrigerator, completely submerge under running water at 70°F or less, or thaw as part of the cooking process.

- Hot foods should be held at 135°F or above and cold foods held at 41°F or below.

- Leftover hot cooked foods must be cooled from 135° to 70°F within 2 hours; from 70° to 41°F within 4 hours. Hot cooked foods can be cooled by placing in shallow pans and using rapid cooling methods (ice bath or blast chiller).

- Wet wiping cloths used for counter tops should be free of food debris and visible soil and should be stored in a solution with chemical sanitizer at proper concentration.

Hazard Analysis Critical Control Point (HACCP)

The *Food Code* also emphasizes use of Hazard Analysis Critical Control Point (HACCP) methods to prevent or reduce risk of potential food safety problems. The seven basic steps in HACCP are:

- Identify hazards (biological, chemical, and/or physical) and assess level of risk.

- Identify the critical control points (CCP)—a point or procedure where loss of control may result in an unacceptable health risk.

- Establish critical limits for preventive measures (time and end-point cooking temperatures).

- Establish procedures to monitor CCPs.

- Establish corrective actions to be taken when a critical limit has been exceeded.

- Establish effective record-keeping systems to document HAACP system.

- Establish procedures to verify that the system is working.

Several segments of the food industry are required to use HACCP programs in food processing. FDA regulates HACCP for the seafood industry and for companies that process fruit and vegetable juices and juice products. The Food Safety and Inspection Service (FSIS) of the U.S. Department of Agriculture regulates HACCP for meat and poultry processors. FDA encourages foodservice establishments to adopt a HACCP system and has published a guide for this purpose. Beginning in the 2005-2006 year, all schools participating in the National School Lunch Program and/or National School Breakfast Program were required by federal law to develop a food safety program that complies with HACCP principles.

Consumer Food Safety

While the *Food Code* serves as a guide for foodservice establishments outside the home, other food safety education materials have been developed to educate consumers about food safety. The Partnership for Food Safety Education, which includes the U.S. Food and Drug Administration, U.S. Department of Agriculture, Centers for Disease Control, National Restaurant Association Educational Foundation, International Food Information Council, Institute of Food Technologists, Academy of Nutrition and Dietetics, and 19 other professional and trade associations developed the Fight Bac campaign in 1997. Fight Bac (www.fightbac.org) divides consumer food safety education into four main areas:

- Clean: focuses on personal hygiene and cleaning of kitchen counters, utensils, equipment, and raw fruits and vegetables.

- Separate: advises consumers to avoid cross-contamination between potentially hazardous foods, hands, and equipment.

- Chill: emphasizes chilling foods promptly and properly.

- Cook: focuses on cooking foods and holding foods at appropriate temperatures.

Source: Partnership for Food Safety Information

CHAPTER 2: Glossary of Food Science Terms

Acid	Substances that furnish hydrogen ions
Acidulate	To make sour or acidic by adding vinegar, lemon juice, or cream of tartar
Aebleskiver	Danish pancake, often filled with apple bits, baked in a special pan so it forms a ball about two inches in diameter
A la carte	Menu in which each dish is ordered and priced separately
A la king	Style of presentation in which food is mixed with a seasoned cream sauce
A la lyonnaise	Cooked or garnished with shredded and fried onions in the style of Lyon, France
A la mode	Made or served in a specific style, such as pie with ice cream
Albondigas (*Spanish)*	Meatball
Albumen	Water-soluble proteins that can be found in egg whites, milk, blood serum, and many other animal and plant tissues
Al dente (*Italian)*	Cooking "to the tooth," a slightly firm but tender stage at which pasta, rice, or vegetables are cooked
Alkali	Substances that form hydroxyl ions that can neutralize an acid
Amandine	Containing or topped with almonds
Andouille (*French)*	A reddish pink sausage made from pork gastrointestinal portions and other ingredients
Anthocyanins	Pigments (classified as flavonoids) that are responsible for the red/blue colors found in certain vegetables and fruits. They are red in the presence of acid; blue-green in the presence of alkali; water soluble
Anthoxanthins	Pigments (classified as flavonoids) that are white in acid, but turn yellow in the presence of alkali; water soluble
Antioxidant	A substance that inhibits the chemical reaction that causes oxidation
Antipasto (*Italian)*	Assorted relishes
AP	As purchased; weight before any trimming or other preparation
AS	As sold or served; weight of an item after processing and/or cooking
Ascorbic acid	Vitamin C; a vitamin that can be used to inhibit enzymatic browning of light-colored fruit such as apples, pears, and bananas; an antioxidant
Au gratin	Sprinkled with crumbs and/or cheese and baked until brown

Au jus	Served with natural juice or gravy
Bagel	Doughnut-shaped roll that is cooked in water before being baked
Bain-marie	Large pan partially filled with boiling water so smaller containers of food can be cooked more slowly; also water bath or can refer to a double boiler
Bake	To cook in an oven or oven-type appliance. When applied to meats in uncovered containers, it is generally called roasting
Baklava	Mid-Eastern confection made of multi-layers of phyllo, honey, and chopped nuts
Bannock	Bread of oat or barley flour, frequently unleavened, and baked in flat loaves; common in the northern British Isles; in New England it is a thin corn bread, baked on a griddle
Barbecue	To roast slowly on a rack or spit over coals or under free flame or an electric heat unit. The food is often brushed with a sauce during cooking
Baste	To moisten meat or other foods during cooking to add flavor and to prevent drying of the surface. The liquid is usually melted fat, meat drippings, fruit juice, sauce, or water
Batch cooking	Dividing estimated amount needed into smaller quantities and cooking as required to meet demand
Batter	A mixture made of flour, liquid, and other ingredients that can be stirred or poured
Béarnaise sauce *(French)*	Sauce made with egg yolks and butter
Beat	To apply rapid, regular motions using a wire whisk, spoon, hand beater, or mixer to a mixture
Béchamel *(French)*	A basic white sauce usually made with milk and sometime stock
Beignet *(French)*	Variety of fritters fried in deep fat
Beurre manie	Thickener composed of equal parts of butter and flour
Bisque *(French)*	A thick, rich, creamy soup
Blanch	To briefly heat vegetables or fruit in steam or boiling water to loosen or remove skins or to inactivate enzymes prior to freezing or drying
Blanquette *(French)*	A stew of light-colored meat or poultry in which the meat is cooked in water without browning
Blend	To mix two or more ingredients thoroughly
Blind-baking	Baking pastry or pastry case without the filling; pre-baking

Blini (*Russian, Polish*)   Small buckwheat crepe usually served with caviar or sour cream

Blintz (*Jewish*)   Thin crêpe with fruit or cheese filling, rolled and sauteed in butter

Boil   To cook in water that is at boiling temperature. Bubbles will rise continually and break on the surface

Boiling point   The temperature at which the atmospheric pressure just exceeds the vapor pressure of a liquid (212°F or 100°C)

Bombe (*French*)   Rich elaborate dessert made of ices, whipped cream, custard, and/or fruit frozen in a melon mold

Borscht (*Russian/ Polish*)   Thick soup made with a beet base, which may contain other vegetables, meat, and a topping of sour cream

Bouillabaisse (*French*)   Thick, hearty soup made from an assortment of fish; originally made in the Mediterranean region of France

Bouillon (*French*)   Broth or clear soup made from various meats, fish, poultry, or vegetables

Bouquet garni (*French*)   Combination of herbs, usually thyme, bay leaf, and parsley, tied together and used as flavoring

Bourguignonne (*French*)   In Burgundy style, braised with red wine, vegetables (mushrooms, onions, carrots), and herbs (parsley, thyme, etc.); could include bacon

Braise   To cook meat or poultry over low heat in a covered utensil in a small amount of liquid or in steam

Bratwurst (*German*)   Brat means chopped meat and wurst means sausage; made from beef, pork, or veal, or combination

Bread   To coat a food with bread or cracker crumbs or other food. The surface may first be coated with a beaten egg or other liquid

Brine   To soak pickled, fermented, or cured foods in a strong salt solution to add flavor and inhibit microbial growth

Brioche   Rich, classic French yeast dough, usually shaped with a topknot

Broil   To cook by direct heat on a rack or spit

Brown   To cook food with moderate or high heat until it browns in color

Browning reactions   Darkening of foods caused by enzymes (light-colored cut fruit or vegetables) or reactions of protein and sugar (baked goods)

Brunoise   A fine dice made of julienne or matchstick cuts that are cut crosswise (1/8" x 1/8" x 1/8")

Buffet	A display of a variety of foods (could be table, serving cart, etc.)
Bulgur	Cracked wheat originating in the Middle East; available as fine, medium, or coarse
Cacciatore *(Italian)*	Food stewed with tomatoes, onion, and garlic
Café au lait *(French)*	Beverage composed of equal parts of strong coffee and heated milk poured simultaneously into the cup
Café noir *(French)*	Black coffee
Caldo *(Spanish)*	A broth, soup, stock, or gravy. In Mexico the term is broader and is used to describe soups or stews with meat and vegetables
Calibrate	Confirmation of a measurement with an established standard
Calorie	See kilocalorie
Canapé *(French)*	Toasted, buttered bread spread or topped with appetizers, flavored spreads, vegetables, or seafood
Candy	To cook fruit or vegetables in sugar or syrup
Cannelloni *(Italian)*	Pasta dish made of squares of dough with meat or cheese filling, filled and baked in a sauce; crêpes sometimes are used instead of pasta
Cannoli *(Italian)*	Cream-filled tubular pastry
Capers	Pickled buds of a Mediterranean shrub with a tart, salty taste, used as a seasoning
Cappuccino *(Italian)*	After-dinner coffee made from hot milk and espresso coffee, flavored with cinnamon
Caramelize	To heat sugar or foods containing sugar until a brown color and characteristic flavor develop
Carte du jour *(French)*	Menu for the day (carte means menu and du jour means of the day [e.g. soup du jour]
Carotenoids	Yellow-to-red pigments found in fruits and vegetables; fat soluble
Cassoulet *(French)*	Stew made from dried beans, assorted meats, and sausages
Caviar	Black caviar is the eggs, or roe, of the sturgeon and is imported from Russia and Iran; red caviar is the roe of salmon
Cellulose	A polysaccharide that provides structural rigidity in cell walls of plants, fruits, and vegetables. It can be softened by cooking but is not digested by humans
Ceviche	Also seviche. Raw fish or seafood marinated in lime juice

Challah	Braided Jewish Sabbath bread
Chantilly *(French)*	Containing whipped cream
Chapatti	Flat bread made from whole wheat, baked on a griddle; from India
Chateaubriand	Thick piece of filet mignon usually prepared for two and served with Béarnaise sauce
Chef or Executive chef	Person in charge of the kitchen; manager responsible for all aspects of food production
Chili con carne	Red beans, tomatoes, meat, and chili pepper seasoning; stew characteristic of southwestern U.S.
Chili rellenos *(Mexican)*	Batter-coated green chili peppers stuffed with mild cheese
Chitterlings	Also chittlins. Well cleaned small intestines of hogs, cut in pieces and boiled, then fried and seasoned
Chop	To cut into pieces with a knife or other sharp tool, blender, or food processor
Chorizo	Hot Spanish or Mexican sausage
Choux *(pâte à choux)*	A light pastry dough made of butter, flour, water, and eggs and used to make profiteroles, croquembouches, éclairs, French crullers, beignets, St. Honoré cake, Indonesian kue sus, and gougères
Chlorophyll	The green pigment in vegetables that turns olive green in the presence of acid and/or heat
Chowder	Thick soup of fish or vegetables and milk
Chutney	Spicy-sweet relish originating in India, popular in England
Cilantro	Pungent herb; also known as Chinese parsley or coriander leaves
Clarify	Make clear by skimming or adding egg white and straining; clarified butter is also known as drawn butter
Coagulation	The change from a fluid state to a thickened curd or clot due to denaturation of protein
Coat	To spread food with or dip it into a substance such as flour or a sauce until it is covered
Coddle	To cook (eggs) in water just below boiling point
Colloidal dispersion	A dispersion of very tiny particles of one substance in another substance; the particles are too large to form a true solution and too small to form a coarse suspension. An example is gelatin dissolved in water

Combine	To stir two or more ingredients together to form a mixture of uniform consistency
Compote	Stewed fruit, often based on dried fruit; a footed bowl
Condiment	Aromatic accompaniment such as pickles, chutney, relishes, and sauces (ketchup, mustards, etc.) usually added by the diner
Consommé	Clarified double-strength brown stock
Controlled atmosphere	A long-term storage technique where respiration of products such as apples is retarded by rigidly controlling temperature and humidity and adding carbon dioxide at a controlled level
Coq au vin *(French)*	Chicken cooked in red wine sauce
Couscous	Pellets of steamed semolina pasta often served with a stew
Couscous *(North African)*	Pasta of crushed and steamed semolina
Cream	To mix one or more foods (usually fat and sugar) with a spoon or mixer until soft and smooth; air is incorporated
Creole *(French)*	Foods containing meat or vegetables with tomatoes, peppers, onions, and other seasonings
Crêpes *(French)*	Very thin pancakes
Croissants *(French)*	A rich, crescent-shaped roll or pastry
Croutons	Small cubes of toasted bread used to garnish soup or salad
Crudités *(French)*	An appetizer of raw vegetables usually served with a dip
Crystallization	The formation of crystals resulting from chemical elements or compounds solidifying in an orderly structure
Cube	To cut food into small squares; to cut the surface of meat in a checkered pattern to increase tenderness
Curdle	To form clots in a smooth liquid (such as milk) by precipitating the protein with heat, acid, or enzymes
Cure	To preserve beef or poultry with a combination of salt or brine, sodium nitrate, and / or nitrite, seasonings, and sometimes smoking. Cured products such as corned beef and ham develop a distinctive pink / red color
Curry	Blend of many spices such as ginger, coriander, cardamom, cayenne, turmeric; originating in India

Cut	To divide food material with a knife or scissors
Cut in	To distribute solid fat throughout dry ingredients using two knives or a pastry blender until flour-coated fat particles are the desired size
Deep fry	To cook food in enough hot fat for submersion or floatation
Dehydration	A method of food preservation where water is removed from food by drying in air, in a vacuum, in inert gas, or by direct application of heat
Demitasse	Small cup of strong, black , after-dinner coffee
Denaturation	A change in the physical structure of protein molecules that alters their characteristics. Heat, for example, denatures the protein of an egg
Dextrinization	Change of starch into smaller, sweeter components with a loss of thickening power by exposure to dry heat
Dice	To cut into small cubes ; small dice = ¼ x ¼ x ¼"; medium dice 3/8 x 3/8 x 3/8" or ½ x ½ x ½"; large dice 5/8 x 5/8 x 5/8" or ¾ x ¾ x ¾"
Dilute	To make less strong by adding liquid
Dissolve	To make a solution such as sugar in water; to melt or liquefy
Dough	A mixture of flour and water (and usually other ingredients) that is still enough to be rolled or kneaded
Drawn	When the entrails of fish or chicken are removed
Drawn butter	See Clarify
Dredge	To cover or coat with flour or other fine substances such as sugar, breadcrumbs, or cornmeal
Du jour *(French)*	"Of the day" used as soup du jour or the soup specialty available that day
Dust	To sprinkle lightly with flour or sugar
Emulsify	To suspend small drops of an immiscible liquid in another, forming an emulsion such as mayonnaise
En Brochette *(French)*	Broiled and served on a skewer
Enchilada *(Mexican)*	Tortilla rolled around meat or cheese filling and covered with sauce
Entrée	In the U.S., the main course; in France, the dish served before the main course
Enzymatic browning	Discolorization of foods, such as cut fruit, due to oxidation catalyzed by enzymes

Enzymes	Proteins that catalyze chemical reactions that change the color, texture, and flavor of foods
EP	Edible portion; weight of item after trimming and preparation
Espagnole	Sauce made of brown stock and flavoring vegetables (i.e., mirepoix and tomatoes) and thickened with a brown roux (also known as brown sauce or Spanish sauce)
Espresso (*Italian*)	Strong, black coffee made with steam
Fabricate	Breaking down a carcass of meat into consumer cuts
Falafel (*Israeli, Middle Eastern*)	Croquettes made of mashed chick peas fried in deep fat
Feijoada (*Brazilian*)	Soup/stew of black beans, meat, and rice
Fermentation	The anaerobic conversion of sugar to carbon dioxide
Fettuccine (*Italian*)	Narrow, flat noodles
Fillet	Strip of boneless lean meat, fish, or poultry
Fines herbes	Equal parts of freshly minced parsley, tarragon, chives, and chervil
Fish sauce	Used in Southeast Asian cuisine. The sauce is made from one type of fish and is often salty. Finger foods are dipped into the sauce
Flake	To break into small pieces, usually with a fork
Flambé	Served after flaming brandy or other high-proof liqueur
Flan	Baked custard with caramel sauce also called crème caramel; also open-faced pastry tart with fruit toppings
Florentine (*Italian*)	Served in the manner of Florence with spinach or a spinach base
Foam	A type of colloidal dispersion in which bubbles of gas are surrounded by liquid
Foie gras (*French*)	Specially fattened goose livers ground to a fine, smooth paste and seasoned
Fold	To combine one ingredient with another by gently turning the mixture with a spoon or spatula to minimize loss of air. Two motions are used: cutting vertically through the mixture and sliding across the bottom of the bowl and up the other side
Fondant	A creamy sugar paste candy or icing
Fondue Bourguignonne (*Swiss*)	Small pieces of meat deep-fried at the table by each diner

Fondue Suisse *(Swiss)*	Melted cheese, white wine and kirsch into which cubes of dry French bread are swirled
Food standards	Specifications for certain foods such as identity, quality, fill of container, and enrichment level that are regulated by governmental agencies
Foo yong	Chinese omelet with bean sprouts, meat, and fish
Frappé *(French)*	Mixture of fruit juices frozen to a slush
Freeze drying	A method of preserving food by first freezing and then drying under a vacuum. The freeze-dried product may be stored without refrigeration and is much lighter in weight than frozen products
Freezing	A method of preserving food by chilling it rapidly at a low temperature
Fricassee	To cook cut pieces of food such as fowl, rabbit, or veal by braising in a sauce
Frijoles refritos *(Mexican)*	Cooked beans that have been mashed and fried
Frittata *(Italian)*	Omelet with flavorful filling or topping
Fritter	Batter-dipped food fried in deep fat or sauteed
Frizzle	To heat or fry until crisp and curled, scored, or seared
Fry	To cook in fat. A small amount of fat is used for pan-frying or sauteing; deep-fat fried foods are submerged in fat
Garde-manger *(French)*	Pantry chef or station responsible for cold food preparation (salads, dressings, charcuterie items, and cold appetizers)
Garnish	To add decorative touches (usually edible) to food that is served
Gazpacho *(Spanish)*	Chilled soup composed of finely chopped raw tomatoes, cucumbers, onions, and other vegetables in spiced tomato juice
Gefilte fish	Also gefullete. German/Jewish stuffed or chopped fish
Gel	A liquid-in-solid colloidal system that does not flow. It can be formed by gelatin, pectin, starch, soured milk, and egg
Gelatinization	The absorption of liquid by starch, which results in swelling of the granules and thickening of the liquid. Heat is required to accomplish this change
Genoise *(French)*	Rich light sponge cake; often used as a base for more elaborate desserts
Ghee *(India)*	A clarified butter

Ginseng	Thick root of plant highly prized in the Orient for its stimulating, refreshing qualities; plant originated in Korea
Glaze	To coat with a glossy mixture that enhances both flavor and appearance of food (such as meats, vegetables, and desserts)
Gluten	The elastic substance formed from manipulating the viscous and insoluble proteins of wheat flour with some liquid
Gnocchi *(Italian)*	Small, tender dumplings made of potatoes, flour, or semolina
Goulash *(Hungarian)*	Beef stew liberally seasoned with paprika
Grate	To produce particles of a specific size by rubbing food (such as carrots or cheese) on a grater (or chopping in a blender or food processor)
Grease	To rub the surface of a pan or dish with fat to prevent food from sticking
Grill	To cook food on a rack with direct heat
Grind	To reduce food to small particles by cutting or crushing mechanically in a grinder, blender, or food processor
Guacamole *(Mexican)*	Smooth paste of avocado, tomato, onion, and green chilis used as an appetizer, salad dressing, and sauce
Gumbo	Thick soup/stew characteristic of Creole cooking in Louisiana; also means okra
Halal *(Arabic)*	"Permissible" object or action permitted under Islamic law (fruits, vegetables, dairy, grains)
Haram *(Arabic)*	"Forbidden" foods containing emulsifiers, enzymes, preservatives, and flavorings that originate in pork or are alcohol-based
Haricot vert *(French)*	Extremely thin, tender variety of green beans which have full flavor when picked young
Hollandaise *(French)*	Thick rich sauce made of egg yolks, butter, and lemon juice
Homogenize	To break up into tiny particles of the same size, such as fat in milk
Hors d'oeuvres	Attractive small appetizers
Huevos *(Spanish)*	Eggs
Hummus	Thick mixture of mashed chickpeas, tahini, oil, garlic, and lemon juice
Hydration	The process of absorbing water

Hydrogenation	The process of adding hydrogen ions to unsaturated (liquid) fat to form a solid or semi-solid fat such as margarine
Hydrolysis	The process of splitting the compounds into simpler components by adding a molecule of water, a reaction that can be facilitated by acid, heat, enzymes, or light
Ice bath	The use of iced water to rapidly cool products
Irradiation	A process in which foods can be exposed to ionizing radiation to lengthen storage life. Depending on dose, irradiation can kill insects, inhibit sprouting, and kill microorganisms
Jardiniere *(French)*	Mixed vegetables in a savory sauce or soup
Julienne	To cut meat, fruit, or vegetables into long, thin strips like matchsticks (1/8 x 1/8 x 2") or fine julienne (1/16 x 1/16 x 2—3") or shoestrings (e.g. shoestring potatoes or fries)
Kabob *(Middle Eastern)*	Also kebob. Skewered pieces of meat and vegetables roasted over flames
Kasha	Russian buckwheat groats; also used in other East European cuisines as a staple
Kilocalorie	The amount of heat required to raise the temperature of 1 kilogram of water (1000 g) 1 degree Celsius
Kim chee *(Korean)*	Spicy fermented cabbage
Kippers	Split, dried, salted, smoked herring; popular English breakfast food
Knead	To work dough by hand or mechanically to develop the gluten needed for structure of baked products
Kobe beef *(Japanese)*	Highly regarded grade of beef from Wagyu cattle raised in Kobe, Japan, with extremely high fat content that is well-marbled throughout
Kolachi *(Middle European)*	Also Kolachy. Yeast roll filled with cheese or preserved fruit
Kosher	Food handled in accordance with Jewish religious customs
Kuchen *(German)*	Cake or coffee cake; also specifically a flat round bread topped with cream cheese and sweetened fruit
Lamination	Dough that has fat incorporated in a series of folds and rolls to form layers producing light, flaky pastry
Lard	To place strips of fat on top of or into gashes in the side of uncooked lean meat or fish to give flavor and prevent drying
Lasagna *(Italian)*	Broad noodles layered with meat, cheese, and sauce

Leading sauce	A basic sauce used in the production of other sauces. Leading hot sauces include Béchamel, Espagnole, Hollandaise, Tomato, and Velouté and leading cold sauces as Mayonnaise and Vinaigrette
Leavening agent	A substance that increases the volume of a baked product (air, steam, and microbiological or chemical agents capable of producing carbon dioxide)
Limpa *(Swedish)*	Rye bread flavored with orange rind
Linguine *(Italian)*	A long, thin and narrow ribbon-like pasta
Luau	Hawaiian feast
Lucia buns *(Swedish)*	Sweet rolls served on St. Lucia Day, December 13
Lukewarm	A temperature of about 95°F (35°C). Lukewarm liquids and foods feel neither hot nor cold when in contact with the inside of the wrist
Macerate	To soak foods in a liquid to soften them and to absorb flavor
Maillard reaction	Dark color resulting from chemical interaction between sugars and proteins when heated (baked goods) or stored together for a long time (dried milk)
Manicotti *(Italian)*	Large tubular noodles stuffed with cheese, meat, or vegetables and served with sauce
Matzos *(Jewish)*	Thin, flat pieces of unleavened bread eaten during Passover
Medallion	Cut of meat, usually from loin or tenderloin, that has a neat, round shape and uniform thickness
Meniscus	The curved upper portion of a liquid that is curved due to surface tension
Menudo *(Mexican)*	Soup / stew made of tripe, hominy, and green chilis
Meringue	A foam of beaten egg whites and sugar that is baked. A soft meringue may be baked on a one-crust pie; a baked, hard meringue is used as a shell for berries or other dessert fillings
Mince	To chop or cut into very small pieces
Minestrone *(Italian)*	Thick vegetable soup
Mirepoix	Mixture of chopped vegetables used in flavoring soup stocks, usually 25% carrots, 50% onions, and 25% celery
Mise en place *(French)*	Preparation, organization, and set up before food production; everything in place
Mix	To combine two or more ingredients into a uniform mixture

Mocha Type of Arabian coffee; also coffee or coffee/chocolate flavored

Moussaka Layers of eggplant alternated with chopped lamb or beef
  (Middle Eastern)

Mousse *(French)* Light delicate dish usually made with gelatin with sweet or savory fillings, depending on the use – sweet for dessert

Nesselrode Dessert or sauce made of candied fruit and chestnuts

Nicoise *(French)* In the style of Nice, meaning use of tomatoes, onions, garlic, capers, and olive oil

Osmosis Movement of water through a semipermeable membrane from an area of low concentration of solute to an area of higher concentration to equalize the osmotic pressure created by differences in concentration

Oven spring Rapid increase in the volume of bread in the first few minutes of baking when yeast hits a hot oven

Paella *(Spanish)* A rice casserole with chicken, seafood, vegetables, and seasonings

Pan-broil To cook uncovered over high heat on a hot surface (usually a fry pan), pouring off accumulating fat

Pan-fry To cook over high heat with a small amount of fat

Panning Cooking vegetables in their own juices and a small amount of fat in a tightly covered pan

Pareve *(Jewish)* In kosher cuisine, foods such as fruits, vegetables, and eggs that may be eaten with either meat or dairy foods

Parboil To boil until partially cooked. Cooking is usually completed by another method

Pare To cut off the outside covering such as skins of vegetables or fruits

Pasta All forms of macaroni products

Pasteurization The process of destroying harmful microorganisms by heating food (such as milk or fruit juice) to a specific temperature and holding for a specific length of time

Pâté *(French)* Ground, seasoned meat or meats served with or without pastry covering

Peel To remove the outer covering of foods such as oranges or bananas

Pesto *(Italian)* Thick pureed mixture of an herb, usually basil, and oil used as a sauce for pasta

Petits fours *(French)* Small fancy iced cakes

pH	A measure of acidity / alkalinity based on the hydrogen ion concentration. On the scale of 1 to 14, 1 is most acidic and 14 is most alkaline. Neutral is a pH of 7
Phyllo	Also Fila, brik, malsouka, yukka. A tissue-thin pastry that is used in the Middle East
Picante	Highly spiced tomato sauce used as a condiment with Mexican foods
Pickling	The process of preserving food by using acid and salt to inhibit microbial growth
Pilaf *(Middle Eastern)*	Also pilou. Browned rice, barley, or cracked wheat variously seasoned
Pinch	The amount of a substance that can be held between the thumb and forefinger; 1/16 teaspoon
Pirozhki *(Russian)*	Small meat-filled pastries used as appetizers
Pit	To remove the seed from whole fruit
Pita	Flat bread with a pocket inside that may be stuffed with meat and/or salad
Poach	To cook in a hot liquid, being careful to retain shape of the food (e.g., poached eggs or fish)
Poi *(Hawaiian and Polynesian)*	Starchy, bland paste made from steamed taro root
Polenta *(Italian)*	Corn meal porridge
Profiteroles	Cream puffs or choux à la crème made of choux pastry ball filled with whipped cream, pastry cream, or ice cream
Proof	In baking, to increase the volume of dough through continued fermentation or to initially test whether yeast is viable
Proteolytic enzymes	Enzymes capable of effecting a chemical reaction that splits proteins into simpler components. Examples are papain (from papaya) and bromelin (from pineapple)
Punch down	To deflate risen yeast dough by pushing it down with the fist
Puree	To press food through a fine sieve or food mill; to blend in a blender or food processor to a smooth, thick mixture; also a thick sauce made from pureed vegetables
Quesadilla *(Mexican)*	Cheese wrapped in a tortilla and heated
Quiche *(French)*	An unsweetened custard frequently containing cheese and usually baked in a pastry shell
Quinoa	A high-protein grain that contains all essential amino acids and is prepared like rice
Ragout *(French)*	Stew made with meat, poultry, or fish, and sometimes vegetables

Rancidity	Flavor and odor deterioration due to either hydrolysis or oxidation of fats
Ratatouille *(French)*	Southern French vegetable stew of onions, tomatoes, zucchini, eggplant, and green peppers
Ravioli *(Italian)*	Filled pasta dough that is boiled and served with a sauce
Reconstitute	To restore concentrated foods such as nonfat dry milk or frozen orange juice to their original form by adding water
Reduce	To decrease volume of liquid by rapidly boiling
Rehydrate	To restore water lost during drying by soaking or cooking dehydrated foods
Rennet	A substance from mammalian, usually stomachs from calves that contains rennin, an enzyme used in cheese making. Also available as vegetable and microbial rennets.
Retrogradation	Formation of crystalline areas of gelatinized starch mixtures (such as bread products and starch pastes) as they age
Rigatoni	Large fluted tubes of Italian pasta, often stuffed and covered with sauce
Rijsttafel	Literally "rice table"; Dutch-Indonesian dinner with rice and an assortment of spicy foods
Risotto *(Italian)*	Wide variety of rice dishes
Roast	To cook uncovered in an oven
Roquefort *(French)*	Blue-veined, pungent cheese; authentic Roquefort comes only from a certain area of France and bears the trademark of a small red outline of a sheep on the label
Roux *(French)*	Mixture of fat and flour used to thicken soups, sauces, and gravies
Salsa	Spanish for sauce. In Mexico, a mixture of chopped fresh tomatoes, peppers, and onions
Sashimi *(Japanese)*	Raw fish served with dipping sauces, usually an appetizer
Sauerbraten *(German)*	Pot roast of beef that has been marinated several days in spicy vinegar sauce
Sauté	To brown or cook in a small amount of fat
Scald	To heat liquid to just below the boiling point; to pour boiling water over food or dip food briefly in boiling water
Scallop	To bake food (usually cut into pieces) with a sauce or other liquid

Score	To cut shallow slits on the surface of meat or food to increase tenderness or to prevent the fat covering from curling
Sear	To brown the surface of foods quickly with high heat
Shred	To cut into thin strips
Sift	Working dry ingredients through a sieve
Simmer	To cook food over low heat in a liquid just below the boiling point (about 180 to 210°F or 80 to 99°C). Bubbles will form slowly and break apart just below the surface
Slurry	A thickener of raw starch and a cold liquid
Smoke point	The temperature at which a fat begins to smoke and emit irritating vapors
Smorgasbord *(Scandinavian)*	Literally "sandwich table"; large assortment of hors d'oeuvres, cold salads, meats, and desserts
Smorrebrod *(Scandinavian)*	Open-face sandwiches, tastefully arranged and garnished
Sol	A fluid colloidal system in which the continuous phase is liquid
Solution	A uniform liquid blend containing a solvent (liquid) and a solute (such as salt or sugar dissolved in the liquid
Sorbet *(French)*	Sherbet made of several kinds of fruits
Soufflé *(French)*	A delicate, baked dish with a base of very thick white sauce and egg yolks blended with whipped egg whites
Sous chef	Chef who is second in command and reports to the executive chef; chef in command of the actual production and minute-to-minute supervision of the staff
Sous vide	Food cooked by vacuum-packing portions into pouches and cooking at precise temperatures in a water bath (immersion circulator, slow cooker, etc.)
Spatzle	Also Spatzen. Small German egg dumplings
Specific gravity	The weight of a specific volume of a substance in relation to the weight of an equal volume of water. At 40° Celsius, 1 milliliter of water weighs 1 gram
Specific heat	The heat or thermal capacity of a substance in relation to that of water
Spumoni *(Italian)*	Rich ice cream containing candied fruit and nuts
Steam	To cook food with steam over boiling water

Steep   To let a food stand in liquid below the boiling point of water to extract flavor or color

Sterilize   To destroy microorganisms by using heat or irradiation

Stew   To simmer food in a liquid

Stir   To mix ingredients with a circular motion

Stir-fry   To fry thinly sliced food quickly in only a little oil, stirring with a tossing motion

Stollen *(German)*   Pastry or yeast coffee cake containing dried and candied fruit and nuts; associated with Christmas

Strain   To remove liquid from food using a strainer

Stroganoff *(Russian)*   A meat mixture with noodles, onions, mushrooms, and a sauce with a sour cream base

Strudel *(Austrian)*   Thin leaves of flaky pastry filled with fruit, cheese, meats or vegetables based on a stretched dough; characteristic of central Europe

Subgum   In Chinese cuisine, meaning mixture of vegetables

Sukiyaki *(Japanese)*   Sauteed beef and vegetables; usually cooked at the table

Supersaturated solution   A solution that contains more solute than an unheated liquid could hold at a given temperature. It is unstable and prone to crystallization

Sushi *(Japanese)*   Appetizer composed of vinegared rice topped with raw fish or wrapped in laver (seaweed ; nori)

Suspension   A substance suspended in a liquid (such as starch in cold water) that will remain combined only when stirred

Syneresis   Drainage of liquid from a gel when cut or disturbed

Table d'hôte *(French)*   In restaurants, a fixed price for all the courses of a meal; opposite of à la carte

Taco *(Mexican)*   Fried tortilla folded around various fillings

Tahini *(Middle Eastern)*   Oily paste prepared by grinding sesame seeds

Tamale *(Mexican)*   Ground corn paste shell wrapped around meat or poultry filling and steamed

Tempura *(Japanese)*   Batter dipped, deep-fried food of any type

Teriyaki *(Japanese)*   Soy sauce marinade used to flavor meat and fish

Timbale   A custard that is cooked in a drum-shaped mold; a pastry shell filled with a creamy mixture

Toast	To brown by direct heat or in a hot oven
Tofu	Soy bean curd used in oriental and vegetarian cooking
Toque *(French)*	Chef's hat (usually white)
Torte	A rich cake usually made of eggs, chopped nuts, and crumbs
Tortilla *(Mexican)*	Thin, unleavened corn bread; in Spain an omelet
Toss	To mix foods lightly with a lifting motion
Tostada *(Mexican)*	Layered salad composed of tortilla, refried beans, shredded lettuce, ground meat, and grated cheese
Trans fat	Formed in the processing of hydrogenated fats; fats with a higher melting point than those in natural cis form
UHT pasteurization	Destroying all harmful microorganisms by high heating of food (138°C for at least 2 seconds) making possible storage in closed sterile container at room temperature or storage for extended periods at refrigerated temperatures
Velouté	Sauce made by thickening white stock with a roux
Vermicelli *(Italian)*	Very narrow type of spaghetti
Vichyssoise *(French)*	Cream soup made with leeks and potatoes; usually served cold
Vinaigrette *(French)*	Marinade or salad dressing of oil, vinegar, pepper, and herbs
Viscosity	The degree to which a fluid flows readily or resists flow
Vol-au-vent *(French)*	Flaky or puff pastry made into a shell
Warm	A temperature of 105 to 115°F (40 to 46°C)
Whey	Protein in milk
Whip	To beat food such as cream, eggs, or gelatin rapidly to incorporate air and increase volume
Wiener schnitzel *(Austrian)*	Vienna style breaded, sautéed veal cutlet
Wonton *(Chinese)*	Squares of noodle dough that are wrapped around meats and vegetables and cooked in boiling water
Yorkshire pudding *(English)*	A batter pudding baked in the drippings of roasting meat

CHAPTER 3: Milk and Milk Products

Milk is the main food for young mammals (not recommended for human infants under age one), and has been used as a food source for people for thousands of years, in countless ways, as food in fluid form and in food products. The term milk usually implies cow's milk in the United States; however, milk from goat, buffalo, and camel are used throughout the world. All milk and milk products should be pasteurized or ultra-pasteurized to destroy pathogenic bacteria (disease-causing bacteria) and meet local ordinances and state standards as well as federal specifications. Nutritional value varies with the type of milk or milk product; calcium, protein, vitamin A, vitamin D, and riboflavin are common nutrients in a variety of milk and milk products. Read the nutrition labels for clarification.

BUTTER

Butter is made from sweet or sour cream and contains not less than 80 percent milkfat. A lactic acid culture may be added to the cream for a short "ripening" period to develop desirable aroma and flavors before the cream is churned. The addition of annatto, a colorant derived from the annatto plant, and salt is optional.

Butter that has been officially graded by the U.S. Department of Agriculture for sale on the retail market bears a shield on the package with a letter grade that indicates the quality of the butter at the time of grading. Grades AA and A are available at the retail level. Grade B is usually used as an ingredient in manufactured applications, rather than sold as a product. Occasionally, the equivalent numerical flavor score of butter is shown under the grade shield. Grades for butter depend on quality factors of flavor, body, texture, color, and salt. The U.S. grade and score relationships are: AA or 93 score, A or 92 score, B or 90 score, and C or 89 score.

Whipped butter has been stirred or whipped to incorporate air or some inert gas to thereby increase the volume and make the butter easier to spread.

STORAGE AND USE

- To store butter, leave it in its original package and keep in a food compartment of the refrigerator or in the freezer.

- Place partially used portions of butter in a covered container, refrigerate, and use within a few days.

- Wrapped in moisture-vapor-proof packaging material, butter can be frozen for up to nine months at 0°F (-18°C).

- To measure butter, press it firmly into individual measuring cups or spoons and level with the straight edge of a spatula. Or measure butter according to these equivalents: 1 lb. = 2 cups = 4 sticks = 32 tablespoons (454 g = 473 ml).

- Whipped butter should not be substituted in most recipes for regular butter or margarine because the volumes are not equivalent.

- To substitute other fats in recipes that call for butter, allow for each cup of butter 1 cup (237 ml) margarine or 7/8 cup (207 ml) hydrogenated shortening or lard plus ½ teaspoon (2.5 ml) salt.

CHEESE

Cheese comes in natural cheese or processed cheese forms, both in a wide variety of flavors, textures, and nutritional value.

NATURAL CHEESE

Cheese is made from cow's, sheep's, or goat's milk or cream and is cured or aged for a specific period of time to develop flavor. It is prepared by precipitating proteins in milk and separating the curd or solid portion from the whey or watery portion. Natural cheese may be classified by texture or consistency and the degree or kind of ripening. Ripening may be obtained through bacteria or mold. Harder cheeses keep longer. Classifications include:

Very hard cheese — Parmesan, Romano, Sap Sago, bacteria- ripened.

Hard cheeses — Cheddar, Colby, Colby Jack, Swiss, and Provolone, bacteria-ripened.

Semisoft to hard cheeses — Edam, Baby Swiss, Gouda, and Feta, bacteria-ripened whey cheeses, unripened.

Semisoft cheeses — Blue (Bleu), Gorgonzola, Roquefort, and Stilton, mold-ripened; Brick, Monterey Jack, and Muenster, bacteria-ripened; mozzarella, unripened.

Soft cheeses — Brie and Camembert, mold-ripened; Limburger, bacteria-ripened; cottage cheese, cream cheese, Neufchatel, and ricotta, unripened.

Grades have been established for cheese such as Cheddar, Colby, Monterey, and Swiss based on specifications for flavor, odor, body, texture, finish, appearance, and color, with additional specifications applicable to cheese of different ages. Swiss cheese is rated for eye formation as well as for flavor, body, and texture. The quality rating of cheese is seldom given in the retail market.

PROCESS CHEESE AND PRODUCTS

Process cheese is a blend of one or more natural cheeses that have been processed using heat to inactivate bacteria and enzymes. Added emulsifiers enhance blending qualities. Included in this group are pasteurized process cheese, process cheese food, process cheese spread, and coldpack cheese, which is not heated.

Pasteurized process cheese has up to 3 percent emulsifying salts such as sodium citrate or disodium phosphate and may contain milk, cream, or whey added to the natural cheese. The maximum moisture content is 40 percent, which is higher than that in the same type of natural cheese.

Cheese food is a product made from a mixture of one or more varieties of cheese with added solids, salt, and up to 3 percent of an emulsifier, all of which are mixed with the aid of heat. The moisture content of a pasteurized cheese food is about 4 percent higher than that permitted for process cheese; the milkfat content is lower. Fruit, vegetables, and meats may be added.

Cheese spreads are similar to cheese foods except that a stabilizer is used, moisture content is about 8 percent more than that in process cheese, and milkfat content is lower. Spreads may be flavored with pimiento, olives, pickles, onion, fruit, vegetables, meats, or other ingredients. Cold pack cheese, or club cheese, is a blend of natural cheeses prepared without heat. Stabilizers, spices, or smoke flavoring often are added. Softer in texture than natural cheese, cold pack cheese spreads readily.

REDUCED-FAT AND LOW SODIUM CHEESE

Reduced-fat cheese may be a natural cheese or a processed cheese. Natural reduced-fat cheese is made from reduced-fat milk and contains less fat and fewer kilocalories than its counterpart. A reduced-fat cheese generally contains more protein and calcium than its full-fat counterpart.

"Light" pasteurized process cheese is made by blending reduced-fat natural cheese with an emulsifier to increase keeping quality and improve melting consistency.

Fat-free cheeses are made from skim milk and cheese cultures. Fat-free ricotta, cottage cheese, and other cheese products are available.

Low sodium cheese contains 140 mg or less sodium per serving. Some varieties are available with two-thirds to one-half less sodium than their regular counterparts.

Imitation cheeses are made from cows' milk that does not meet Federal Standards of Identity for composition.

They may be made from filled milk or mixtures of sodium and calcium caseinate, emulsifying salts, flavorings, and vitamins and minerals.

STORAGE AND USE

- All cheese keeps best at refrigerator temperatures of 35 to 40°F (2–4°C). Store in the original wrap or container until opened, and then rewrap cheese tightly in plastic wrap or place in a clean, airtight container.

- Cheese should be used by the date listed on the container or wrapper.

- Uncreamed dry curd cottage cheese may be frozen in appropriate freezer containers. It will keep well for about a month. Textural changes may occur.

- Most hard cheeses can be frozen for six to eight weeks, but freezing results in a crumbly texture, which is difficult to slice. To freeze cheese, tightly wrap pieces of one pound (454 g) or less and about an inch (2.5 cm) thick in freezer wrap or in moisture-proof, air-tight packaging and freeze at 0°F (-18°C). Thaw cheese in the refrigerator and use within a few days after thawing.

- For full flavor and aroma, serve cheese at room temperature, or 20 to 60 minutes after removal from the refrigerator. The exceptions are soft, unripened cheeses such as cottage, cream, or Neufchatel cheeses, which should be served chilled unless being used as an ingredient in omelets, casseroles, and other hot dishes.

- Cooking temperatures for cheese should be low to prevent stringiness and toughness. High temperatures cause cheese to become leathery, lose flavor, and separate fat.

- Cheese that is thoroughly chilled grates or shreds more easily than cheese at room temperature.

- When mold accumulation is found on cheese, trim at least a 1-inch section of cheese away from the affected area and discard. Use the remaining cheese immediately.

- Reduced-fat cheeses can be added to casseroles, salads, or sandwiches. The low-fat cheese does not "string" and melt as its full-fat counterpart does.

CREAM

Cream is the fat portion of milk that rises to the surface when raw milk is allowed to stand. Most milks with fat are homogenized to stabilize the dispersion of milkfat globules throughout the milk, so the fat does not rise to form a cream layer. The milk is forced under pressure through small apertures that break the fat globules into smaller ones.

Cream may be separated from milk by centrifugal force. To meet Federal Standards of Identity, cream must have not less than 18 percent milkfat. Emulsifiers, stabilizers, sweeteners, flavorings, or other optional ingredients also may be added.

Half-and-half is a mixture of milk and cream with 10.5 to 18 percent milkfat. Half-and-half is usually homogenized.

Light cream is coffee or table cream that is sometimes homogenized. It usually has 20 percent milkfat, but the fat content can range between 18 to 30 percent milkfat.

Light whipping cream contains between 30 and 36 percent milkfat and whips up satisfactorily, but does not freeze successfully.

Heavy cream or whipping cream contains 36 to 40 percent milkfat and is not homogenized. As a foam, it tends to be more stable than light whipping cream foams.

Pressurized whipped cream is whipping cream packed in aerosol cans under pressure. It is made from a mixture of cream, sugar, stabilizers, emulsifiers, flavors, and a gas-forming substance such as nitrous oxide. State regulations specify the kind of cream and minimum fat content. Read the label for percent of fat content.

Dairy sour cream is sweet cream to which a lactic acid culture has been added. Sour cream must comply with individual state requirements for minimum milkfat of the cream used (usually 18 to 20 percent).

Sour half-and-half is made with half-and-half rather than cream, and the acidity is not less that 0.5 percent. Products that resemble sour cream are sour half-and-half dressing and sour cream dressing in which butter or other dairy ingredients replace the cream or milk.

Reduced-fat sour cream is made like dairy sour cream, but skim milk has been added to reduce the fat content. There is also fat-free sour cream available with thickening agents.

Sour cream dressing or sour half-and-half dressing resembles sour cream and sour half-and-half except some of the cream and/or milk is replaced by other dairy ingredients such as butter.

STORAGE AND USE

- Cream should be kept in its original container and refrigerated at 40°F (4°C) or lower until used.

- Cream has a pull date on the package label. The pull date indicates when the product should be withdrawn from retail sale. This date allows for additional storage life when the consumer's refrigerator is maintained at 35 to 40°F (1–4°C). Ultra-pasteurized cream will keep several weeks in the refrigerator. Once opened, it should be treated like pasteurized cream and used within a few days.

- In recipes using sour cream, add the sour cream at the end of the cooking period or combine with flour or condensed soup to help prevent separation or curdling.

MILK

Pasteurized milk has been subjected to temperatures that ensure destruction of pathogenic (disease-causing) microorganisms, some spoilage bacteria, and natural milk enzymes. This results in a prolonged refrigerated shelf life. However, it has not been sterilized. Milks pasteurized by vat, batch (long-time-low-temperature [LTLT], 145°F, 63°C 1800 seconds), high-temperature-short-time [HTST], higher-heat-shorter time [HHST]), or ultra-pasteurization must be refrigerated. Milk pasteurized by ultra-high temperature (UHT) (280–320°F, 138–150°C for 2–6 seconds) and packaged in aseptic containers is shelf stable for about three months. When opened, it must be refrigerated.

FLUID MILKS

Fluid milks are classified primarily by the milkfat content, nonfat milk solids, and added nutrients. Vitamin D is regularly used to fortify most fluid milks—400 International Units (IU) per quart (946 ml). Fluid low fat milk products also may be fortified with vitamin A, which is removed with the milkfat. The vitamin A is added at 2000 IU per quart (946 ml).

	Milkfat %	Milk Solids Not Fat (MSNF) %	Nutrient Added
Whole	>3.25	>8.25	D
Reduced-fat	1.1–2	+8.25	A, D
Low-fat	0.6–1	+8.25	A, D
Fat-free / Skim	<0.2–0.5	+8.25	A, D

Flavored milk includes a variety of chocolate or cocoa flavored products. Other flavors such as strawberry, caramel, coffee, and French vanilla, may be used for flavored milks or drinks. Caloric content of flavored milks or drinks varies according to the amount of milkfat and the composition of other added ingredients. Although a variety of flavors have been added to the market, chocolate remains the most popular. However, one should read the labels because some drinks may have more additives than natural milk ingredients.

Kind of Milk	Milk	Other Flavor	Additives
Chocolate	Whole	Chocolate	Sweetener
Chocolate flavored milk	Whole	Cocoa syrup	Sweetener
Chocolate drink	Fat-free/low-fat	Chocolate	Sweetener
Chocolate flavored drink	Fat-free/low-fat	Cocoa syrup	Sweetener

CULTURED AND SOURED MILKS

Cultured buttermilk is obtained by treating pasteurized skim or part-skim milk with a suitable culture of lactic acid bacteria. The lactic acid produced gives the characteristic acidity and increased thickness of the product.

Buttermilk originally was a byproduct of butter making.

Sour milk is milk soured naturally or artificially by the action of lactic acid bacteria or artificially by the addition of vinegar or lemon juice. Milk that has been soured to the stage that a firm curd has formed is called clabber. The whey and curds have not separated.

Acidophilus cultured milk is prepared by the addition of a Lactobacillus acidophilus concentrated culture to lowfat or skim milk that has been pasteurized, homogenized, and chilled. The rapid chilling halts bacteria growth, retaining the sweet flavor and consistency of the milk.

Bifidobacteria milk, as produced and marketed in the U.S., is a nonfermented, lowfat milk containing 1 percent acidophilus/bifidobacteria culture. Bifid-amended dairy products are in great demand in Japan and Europe. Products fermented with bifidobacteria culture have a mild, acidic flavor, similar to that of yogurt. The culture is added during fermentation or to the finished fermented or fresh product prior to shipment. NOTE: The fat percentages used with milk products are expressed as a percent of weight, not caloric content.

YOGURT

Yogurt is a creamy, custard-like cultured milk product made by fermenting whole, low-fat, or skim milk with a bacterial culture such as Streptococcus thermophilus and Lactobacillus bulgaricus. The minimum amount of milk solids is 8.25 percent with an average of 15 percent solids and 0.5 percent acid. The milkfat standards for lowfat yogurts range from 0.5 to 3 percent; nonfat yogurt contains 0.5 percent or less.

Plain, flavored-containing-no-fruit, and flavored-with fruit yogurts are available. Coffee, vanilla, and lemon are examples of flavored yogurt containing no fruit.

If yogurt contains a fruit it may be sundae-style with fruit on the bottom of the container topped with plain or flavored yogurt, or Swiss- or French-style with fruit blended throughout plain or flavored yogurt.

Frozen yogurt is prepared by adding suitable stabilizers, nonfat milk solids, sweeteners, fruits, and juices to cultured yogurt before freezing. It may be soft or hard. Federal standards have not been established for frozen yogurt.

Low-lactose yogurt has about 60 percent less lactose than milk, making this product suitable for lactose-intolerant people.

Probiotic yogurt contains live microorganisms (e.g., Lactobacillus and Bifidobacterium), which results in a health benefit.

Greek yogurt has made a positive impact on the food market by providing satiety and health value. Initially it is produced similarly to regular yogurt, but contains more protein, more probiotics, and less water.

CONCENTRATED AND DRIED MILK PRODUCTS

Evaporated and evaporated skimmed milk have about 60 percent of the water removed. They may be fortified with vitamins D and/or A. Whole milk concentrates are homogenized. The milk is then sealed in cans and sterilized. According to federal standards, evaporated milk must contain at least 7.5 percent milkfat and not less than 25.5 percent total milk solids. Evaporated skimmed milk must contain not less that 0.5 percent milk fat and a minimum of 20 percent total solids and be fortified with 125 IU of vitamin A per fluid ounce (30 ml). The composition of fats and solids of evaporated milks mixed with an equal volume of water is slightly above the average of fresh milks.

Sweetened condensed milk and sweetened condensed skimmed milk are the products resulting from the evaporation of about half the water from whole or skimmed milk, and the addition of refined cane and/or corn sugar in amounts (44 percent) sufficient for preservation. Therefore, this form of canned milk has not been sterilized. The high sugar adds to the browning of the milk when heated. The high concentration of milk protein allows thickening with the addition of acid or heat to make toppings or desserts.

Ultrahigh-Temperature Milk (UHT) can be stored on shelves without being refrigerated for months (but must be refrigerated after opening). The laminated aseptic cartons provide milk that is ideal for situations (camping, hiking, etc.) in which refrigeration is not an option.

Dried whole milk is similar to fresh whole milk but it is packed in vacuum-packed or gas-packed containers to prevent deterioration. It contains not less than 26 percent milk fat and not more than 4 percent moisture. U.S. grades are Extra and Standard with dry whole milk also having a Premium grade.

Nonfat dry milk is the product resulting from the removal of fat and water from pasteurized milk. It contains not over 5 percent moisture and 1.5 percent milkfat by weight. Nonfat dry milk contains the same relative proportions of proteins, minerals, and water soluble vitamins as fluid nonfat milk and it is fortified with vitamins A and D. Most nonfat dry milk is instantized to form rather coarse, creamy-white, free-flowing particles that dissolve readily in water.

SPECIALTY MILKS

Reduced-lactose or lactase-treated milk is pasteurized milk to which lactase, an enzyme, is added. The lactase hydrolyzes lactose to glucose and galactose. Lactose-intolerant individuals can use lactase-treated milk or purchase lactase tablets to add to milk.

Low sodium milk is a product that has about 95 percent of the sodium replaced with potassium by an ion exchange method resulting in about 6 mg of sodium per cup (237 ml) as compared to 120 mg in regular milk. Both fresh or canned low sodium milk may be available.

Kefir and koumiss are fermented milk beverages commonly produced in Southwestern Asia and similar in taste to yogurt. They are prepared by using kefir grains, which contain bacteria, and a lactose-fermenting yeast held together by layers of coagulated protein. Acid production is controlled by the bacteria, while yeast produces alcohol and some carbon dioxide. The final concentration of lactic acid is 0.8 percent, and alcohol may be as high as 1 percent.

Eggnog is made from pasteurized milk or cream, pasteurized eggs, and sugar, and is flavored with vanilla. It is commonly available during November and December.

STORAGE AND USE

- Use milk in order of pull date found on the container.

- Yogurt keeps about 10 days after the pull date stamped on the carton.

- Unopened packages of any shelf-stable milk should be stored in a cool, dry place. After opening, the unused milk must be refrigerated.

- Evaporated milks may be substituted for other milks. Sweetened condensed milk, however, is not a satisfactory substitute because of the high sugar content that affects flavor and texture.

- To measure dry milk, pour from package or spoon lightly into individual measuring cup, heaping to the brim. Level with the straight edge of a spatula or knife. Shaking the cup to level the powder tends to pack it down and gives an inaccurate measure.

- In recipes, dry milk may be added either to dry or liquid ingredients unless the recipe specifically calls for reconstitution.

- For best flavor, milk for drinking should be served icy cold from the refrigerator. Store milk in its original container.

- Use of acidophilus milk in cooking will destroy the culture.

FROZEN DAIRY PRODUCTS

Ice cream is made from a pasteurized mixture of milk, cream, sugar, stabilizers, flavorings, and sometimes eggs. Coloring also may be added. As the mixture is frozen, it is whipped to approximately 80 to 100 percent more than its original volume. The finished product usually weighs about 4.5 pounds per gallon (2 kg/3.7l) and contains not less than 1.6 pounds (726 g) of food solids per gallon (3.7l). The milkfat content ranges from 8 to 14 percent, usually 10 to 12 percent for plain vanilla ice cream, although some special ice creams may be as high as 20 percent.

Federal standards require that plain vanilla ice cream contain at least 10 percent milkfat and 20 percent total milk solids by weight. Ice cream with chocolate, nuts, or fruits must contain at least 8 percent milkfat and 16 percent total milk solids.

Frozen custard and French custard ice cream are products with high levels of egg yolk solids cooked as a custard before freezing.

Ice milk is a product made in the same manner and with the same ingredients as ice cream, but the ingredients are present in different proportions. The milkfat content ranges from 2 to about 7 percent and the total milk solids must be at least 11 percent, according to the federal standard. It may be either soft- or hard-frozen drawn from the freezer.

Sherbet is a frozen product made of a pasteurized mixture of sugar, milk solids, stabilizer, flavorings such as fruit, fruit juices, or extract, and water. Milk fat content of sherbet is 1 to 2 percent, and the total milk solids content is 2 to 5 percent.

Refrigerated puddings are made with whole or skim milk, packaged and held at refrigeration temperatures in the grocery store and at home.

STORAGE AND USE

- Store ice cream in a tightly closed container at 0°F (-18°C) for up to two months.

- For easy serving, remove frozen dairy products from freezer to refrigerator 10 minutes before serving.

- Ice crystals can be minimized by covering the product with plastic wrap before closing. Small crystals also are retained if the mixture is not allowed to freeze.

WHIPPING PROPERTIES

Cream — When whipped, cream increases two to three times in volume depending on the type of beater used. The fat content should be 30 to 40 percent. Pasteurization and homogenization decrease foam volume and stability. Cream chilled for 48 hours has increased foam volume and stability.

- To whip cream, chill utensils (50°F, 10°C) before use. Keep utensils and cream cold during preparation. Choose a deep bowl just wide enough for beater. Add sugar after whipping, never before. Beat rapidly until stiff, but do not over beat or butter flakes will be formed.

- Whipped cream should be kept chilled at 50°F (10°C) or below until used. The foam is stable for about one hour.

- Whipped cream freezes well, particularly in individual serving portions. Once the portions are frozen, wrap in moisture-proof, airtight packaging and keep frozen until used.

Evaporated milk — Evaporated milk, when whipped, increases two to three times in volume. The foam is less stable than whipped cream unless the milk is made acid or supplemented with gelatin.

- Undiluted evaporated milk will whip best if it is first chilled below 32°F (0°C) until fine ice crystals form.

- To stabilize the foam, increase the acidity by adding 1 tablespoon (15 ml) lemon juice or vinegar for each cup (250 ml) of undiluted evaporated milk. Whip the milk and then fold in the juice or soften ½ teaspoon (2.5 ml) unflavored gelatin in 2 teaspoons (10 ml) cold water and dissolve in 1 cup (250 ml) scalded undiluted evaporated milk. Chill as above, whip, sprinkle with ¼ cup (60 ml) powdered sugar, and fold in.

Nonfat dry milk — Nonfat dry milk triples in volume when whipped and is stable for several hours.

- Use ⅓ cup (80 ml) cold water to ½ cup (125 ml) instant nonfat dry milk. Chill and whip until the mixture is thick enough to stand in soft peaks. Add 1 tablespoon (15 ml) lemon juice and continue to whip until stiff peaks form. Then beat in 2 to 4 tablespoons (30– 60 ml) powdered sugar.

- Whipped nonfat dry milk should be refrigerated and kept chilled until served.

CHAPTER 4: Meat

Meat is generally defined as the edible portions of cattle, swine, and sheep. The major physical component of meat as it appears in the market is lean muscle tissue. Depending on the cut of meat, adipose tissue (fat), connective tissue, and skeletal tissue (bone) also may be present.

The most abundant component of meat is water, which ranges from 45 to 75 percent. The amount of water in the tissues, which decreases as the animal ages and deposits fat, affects the texture, color, and flavor of the muscle.

High quality proteins are abundant in all muscle tissue. Different proteins behave in various ways during food preparation. Some toughen; others become tenderer during cooking.

The amount of fat varies with the species, the particular animal, and the cut. Protein is important for building and repairing body tissue. The amount of adipose tissue differs widely among animals. As the animal grows and ages, subcutaneous fat is deposited just beneath the skin and abdominal fat is deposited around the kidney and in the pelvic area. Then fat is deposited between the muscles (intermuscular or seam fat). Finally, fat is deposited within the muscles (intramuscular fat or marbling).

Other important nutrients in meat that occur in significant amounts are minerals (iron, phosphorous, zinc) and most of the B vitamin complex (thiamin, riboflavin, niacin, B6, and B12). Vitamin B12, essential for growth and the synthesis of DNA, occurs naturally only in animal foods.

Meat is marketed in many forms: fresh, frozen, freeze-dried, canned, cured, smoked, dried, and cured and smoked. Many meat items are available both raw and cooked.

FRESH MEAT

BEEF

The major sources of beef on the retail market are from:

Steers — male animals that have been castrated as calves. Steers (15 to 24 months old) account for more than ⅔ of the high-grade beef on the market.

Heifers — young female animals that have not borne calves. Heifers produce high grade meat.

Cows — female cattle that have borne one or more calves.

Bullocks — young bulls less than two years of age that have begun to develop secondary characteristics of a bull.

Veal — a form of immature cow less than four months of age. It contains little fat.

Calf — is meat from immature cattle, about four to nine months old. Calves weighing 400 to 800 pounds (181 to 363 kg) at the time of slaughter are classified as "baby beef."

LAMB

Meat from sheep less than one year of age accounts for about 90 percent of the lamb on the market. Lamb is designated as:

Spring Lambs — lambs from three to seven months, weighing 70 to 120 pounds (32–54 kg).

Yearlings — sheep approximately one to two years of age.

Mutton — meat from sheep that are older than two years.

PORK

Most pork is from young swine of either sex less than one year of age. Most of the pork on the retail market is from:

Pigs — swine that are less than four months of age and/or weigh less than 120 pounds (54 kg).

Hogs — swine that are more than four months of age and weigh more than 120 pounds (54 kg).

Barrows — male swine castrated when young.

Gilts — female swine that have not had offspring or have not reached an evident stage of pregnancy.

Although most beef, lamb, and veal cuts are sold fresh, much pork is also available in cured or cured and smoked forms. See Table 4.1 for the location and bone shape of various retail cuts of beef, veal, lamb, and pork.

VARIETY MEATS

Organ meats from beef, veal, pork, and lamb are excellent sources of many essential nutrients. They include: brains, heart, kidneys, liver, tongue, tripe (stomach tissue), and sweetbreads (thymus). Many cultures appreciate these highly nutritive cuts as a part of their diet (British and Canadian kidney pie, Scottish haggis, French pâté, etc.).

PROCESSED MEAT

Processed meat may be defined as meat that has been changed by any mechanical, chemical, or enzymatic treatment, which alters the taste, appearance, or keeping quality of the product. It is made from wholesome meat that has been inspected at every stage of production. Major categories are:

SAUSAGE

Seasoned chopped meat may be sold in bulk or as stuffed links, with casings of natural or synthetic materials. Trimmings and some of the less popular meat cuts from pork, beef, veal, lamb, poultry, or a combination of these meats may be used in the processing of sausage.

More than 200 varieties of sausages and cold cuts are marketed in the United States. Some sausages are made from meat that is cured, smoked, cooked, or treated by a combination of these processes. Others may be finely or coarsely textured, fermented, dried, or semi-dried. Sausages are classified as:

Fresh — sausages made from ground meat and not cured, smoked, or cooked. They must be cooked before serving. Examples are fresh pork sausage, fresh bratwurst, chorizo, and Italian-style sausage.

Uncooked and Smoked — sausages that are smoked after forming and must be cooked before serving. Examples are smoked pork sausage, kielbasa, and smoked country-style sausage.

Cooked — sausages that have been cured and cooked. They are ready-to-eat, but may be heated before serving. Blood sausage, precooked bratwurst, liverwurst, and braunschweiger are some examples.

Cooked and Smoked — products made from meat that has been cured, formed into sausages, cooked, and lightly smoked. They are ready-to-eat, but may be heated before serving. Examples are cotto salami, bologna, frankfurters, and Vienna sausage.

Dry and Semi-Dry — sausages that may be smoked or unsmoked. Processing always includes curing and generally involves cooking at the plant. Carefully controlled fermentation acts as a preservative and provides the distinctive flavors. Hard salami is usually a dry sausage, while summer sausage is semi-dry. Cervelat, thuringer, pepperoni, and mortadella are examples of these ready-to-eat sausages.

TABLE 4.1

IDENTIFICATION OF MEAT CUTS[1]

Location	Beef	Veal	Lamb	Pork
Breast and forelegs	Brisket Shank Cross Cuts Short Plate	Breast Riblets Shank Cross Cuts	Breast Breast, rolled Riblets Spareribs Shanks	Spareribs Bacon Salt Pork
Shoulder/ Chuck	Arm Steak or Pot Roast	Arm Steak or Roast	Arm Chops or Roast	Arm Steak or Arm
	Blade Steak or Roast	Blade Steak or Roast	Blade Chops or Roast	Picnic Roast
	Chuck Eye Steak or Roast		Shoulder Roast	Blade Steak
	7-bone Steak or Pot Roast		Neck Slices	Blade Boston
	Short Ribs			Boston Butt
	Shoulder Steak or Pot Roast			
Rib	Rib Steak or Roast, small end	Rib Chops or Roast	Rib Chops or Roast	Rib Chops
	Rib Roast, large end	Crown Roast	Crown Roast	Center Rib Roast
	Rib Eye Steak or Roast			
Loin (Short Loin)	Cube Steak	Loin Chops or Roast	Double Loin Chops	Loin Blade Chops or Roast
	Top Loin Steak or Roast	Loin Kidney Chops	Loin Chops or Roast	Loin Chops
	Tenderloin Steak or Roast (Filet Mignon)	Top Loin Roast		Center Loin Roast
	T-Bone Steak			Tenderloin
	Porterhouse Steak			Top Loin Chops or Roast
				Canadian Bacon
				Country-Style Ribs
				Backribs

IDENTIFICATION OF MEAT CUTS[1] (CONTINUED)

Location	Beef	Veal	Lamb	Pork
Sirloin	Sirloin Steak flat, pin, round or wedge bone Sirloin Roast Top Sirloin Steak	Sirloin Steak or Roast	Sirloin Chops or Roast	Sirloin Chops or Roast Sirloin Cutlets
Leg (Ham/ Round)	Bottom Round Steak or Roast	Round Steak or Roast	Leg, Leg Slice or Roast	Ham Steak or Leg (Fresh Ham) Roast
	Eye Round Steak or Roast	Rump Roast		Leg (Fresh Ham)
	Top Round Steak or Roast	Cutlets		Center Slice
	Rump Steak			
	Rump Roast			
	Round Tip Steak or Roast			
Flank	Flank Steak			

[1] Location of bone of retail cuts of meat are often clues to identification.

CUT	BONE
HIP (SIRLOIN)	Pin bone (near short loin) Flat bone (center cuts) Wedge bone (near round)
LEG OR ROUND	Leg or round bone
BREAST OR BRISKET	Breast and rib bones

CUT	BONE
SHOULDER ARM	Arm bone
SHOULDER BLADE	Blade bone (near neck) Blade bone (center cuts) Blade bone (near rib)
RIB	Back bone and rib bone
SHORT LOIN	Back bone (T-shape) T-bone

From: Amy Brown. *Understanding Food: Principles & Preparation*, 4th ed. Wadsworth, 2011.

Specialty Meats — meats that are cured and fully cooked during processing and are ready-to-eat. Loaf examples are honey, minced ham, old-fashioned, olive, pepper, and pickle and pimiento.

CURED WHOLE MUSCLE CUTS

Curing and drying are among the oldest methods of preserving meats. Salt, sugar, nitrites, and nitrates all may be used in the curing process. Salt acts as a preservative and a flavor enhancer; sugar also improves the flavor. Today, nitrites are the primary curing ingredient used in meat products. Nitrites develop the characteristic red-pink color in the lean parts of meat, impart a typically cured flavor, and inhibit the growth of a number of food poisoning and spoilage microorganisms, including *Clostridium botulinum*. Cured whole muscle cuts include:

Ham — the hind leg of pork that has been cured and smoked or cured and canned. One of the most highly valued pork products, ham can be produced three ways: bone-in, semi-boneless, and boneless. There are also cooked and uncooked varieties. To be labeled "fully cooked," hams must be cooked to an internal temperature of 148°F (65°C) at the processing plant. No additional heating is necessary for fully cooked hams. To serve warm, however, ham should be cooked to 130 to 140°F (55–60° C) for optimum palatability. Hams that are labeled "cook-before eating" must be cooked to an internal temperature of 160 to 170° F (71–77° C) before serving.

Country-style hams — specialty hams that have been dry-cured, smoked, and aged to provide a distinct flavor and texture. Before baking, these hams require soaking or simmering.

Corned (Cured) Beef — prepared from brisket or round. Formerly, "corning" referred to preserving meat by sprinkling it with grains ("corns") of salt. Today, corned beef is cured with a pickle solution of water, salt, sugar, nitrite, and spices.

Bacon — produced primarily from pork bellies. Beef bacon is made from boneless beef short plate, which is similar to the belly in pork. Canadian-style bacon is made from the top loin muscle of pork, usually from heavier hogs. Both bacon and Canadian bacon are cured and smoked.

Dried Beef — made from the round that has been cured, lightly smoked, and dried.

Pastrami — made from beef brisket, plate, or top round. After dry-curing with salt, the beef is rubbed with a paste of garlic powder, ground cumin, red pepper, cinnamon, cloves, and allspice. It is then smoked and cooked.

Pork Shoulder — can be divided into two major cuts: Picnic (arm) and Boston (blade). They can be prepared by the same methods used for hams. Shoulder cuts are usually priced more economically than leg cuts, due to differences in palatability and yield of edible portion.

RESTRUCTURED MEAT

Restructured meat products are generally made from flaked, ground, or sectioned beef or pork, which is then shaped into roasts, steaks, or loaves. The restructuring process consists of three steps: reducing or modifying the particle size, blending, and reforming into the desired shape. Examples of restructured meats are smoked sliced beef and most boneless hams.

INSPECTION PROGRAMS

The Federal Meat Inspection Act of 1906 made inspection mandatory for all meat that was transported across state lines. The Wholesome Meat Act of 1967 required that inspection of meat sold within a state meet requirements at least as stringent as those of the federal system. Federal meat inspection is the responsibility of the Food Safety and Inspection Service, a division of the U. S. Department of Agriculture (USDA). State inspection is the responsibility of each state government, with partial funding by the federal government. These federal and state inspection programs ensure that only healthy animals are used for meat and guarantee that facilities and equipment meet sanitation standards. The Meat Inspection Program also includes inspection of meat at various stages of processing; temperature monitoring for both fresh and cooked meat; review of packaging and labels; control and monitoring the use of additives; and control and monitoring of imported meat.

To be designated as kosher ("fit and proper"), meat must be processed under the supervision of persons authorized by the Jewish faith and must meet the standards of the Mosaic and Talmudic laws. To be designated as halal ("lawful" or "permitted"), meat must be slaughtered according to Muslim laws.

MEAT GRADES

The USDA meat-grading system that is used in buying and selling most meat was established in 1927; it sets standards of quality and yield of edible meat. USDA administers the program, but participation is voluntary. There are federal grades for beef, veal, lamb, and pork; however, there are more grades for beef than for other meats due to the greater variance in age and weight of the animals. A shield-shaped purple stamp indicates the USDA quality grade. In addition, individual packers and retailers may use their own brand names to designate different grade of meat. Federal designations are:

Beef — Prime, Choice, Select, Standard, Commercial, Utility, Cutter, and Canner. The last four grades are seldom sold in retail stores. Beef carcasses also may be yield-graded according to the predicted percentage of edible meat. The range is from one (highest yield) to five (lowest yield).

Veal and Lamb — Prime, Choice, Good, Standard, Utility, and Cull. There is no Standard grade for lamb. Only lamb may be yield-graded from U.S. No. 1 (highest yield) to U.S. No. 5 (lowest yield).

Pork — U.S. No. 1, U.S. No. 2, U.S. No. 3, and U.S. No. 4. The basis for grading pork is the cutability of the carcass and the quality of the meat. The range is from U.S. No. 1 (highest yield) to U.S. No. 4 (lowest yield).

MEAT STORAGE AND USE

Proper storage is essential for maintaining food safety and quality. When meat spoils, the color, odor, and texture deteriorate. When food is contaminated it is invaded by microorganisms, which may not be detected by an off odor or color, but can cause food poisoning and infections in humans. Fortunately, most bacteria that can cause food poisoning cannot grow at low refrigerator temperatures. Meat must always be kept refrigerated before and after cooking or serving. Recommended storage time for maximum quality of meats at refrigerator and freezer temperatures are shown in Table 4.2. The following are a few guidelines for safe meat storage.

- Fresh meat should be stored in the coldest part of the refrigerator and used within a few days. The temperature should be as low as possible, approximately 36 to 40°F (2 –4° C).

- Meat can be kept in the original supermarket wrap in the refrigerator for several days or in the freezer for up to two weeks.

- For longer freezer storage, meat should be tightly rewrapped in moisture-vapor-proof material designed for freezer use (e.g., foil, freezer paper, and some transparent wraps and food storage bags). Be sure to label and date the packages and store at 0° F (-18°C) or lower.

- Cured meats can be refrigerated in the original wrapper, but should be used within one or two weeks.

- Unopened canned hams can be refrigerated until ready to use, unless the label indicates otherwise.

- Cooked meats should be wrapped or placed in tightly covered dishes or containers and refrigerated within two hours after serving.

- To defrost frozen meat, keep it wrapped, and let it stand in the refrigerator. Thaw time will depend on size and thickness of the cut—approximately 4 to 7 hours per pound (0.5 kg) for large roasts, 3 to 5 hours per pound (0.5 kg) for a small roast, and 12 to 14 hours for a 1-inch (2.5 cm) thick steak. Thawed meat can be refrozen if the temperature of the meat has not risen above 40°F (4°C).

TABLE 4.2
REFRIGERATOR AND FREEZER STORAGE TIMETABLE

Meat	Cut	Refrigerator 36° to 40° F (2-4° C)	Freezer 0° F or Colder (-18° C)
Fresh	Beef Cuts	3 to 4 days	6 to 12 months
	Veal Cuts	1 to 2 days	6 to 9 month
	Pork Cuts	2 to 3 days	6 months
	Lamb Cuts	3 to 5 days	6 to 9 months
	Ground Beef, Veal and Lamb	1 to 2 days	3 to 4 months
	Ground Pork	1 to 2 days	1 to 3 months
	Variety Meats	1 to 2 days	3 to 4 months
	Leftover Cooked Meats	3 to 4 days	2 to 3 months
Processed	Luncheon Meats**	3 to 5 days	1 to 2 months
	Sausage, fresh pork**	2 to 3 days	1 to 2 months
	Sausage, smoked**	1 week	1 to 2 months
	Sausage, dry and semi-dry (unsliced)	2 to 3 days	1 to 2 months
	Frankfurters*	3 to 5 days	1 to 2 months
	Bacon**	1 week	1 to 2 months
	Smoked Ham, whole	1 week	1 month
	Ham Slices**	3 to 4 days	1 to 2 months

* Meat in freezer wrapping.

** If vacuum packaged, check manufacturer's date.

COOKING METHODS

Heat affects the physical properties of meat by making it or keeping it tender, flavorful, and safe to eat. Different cooking methods are used to maximize the flavor and eating enjoyment of various cuts of meat. When heat is applied to meat, two changes occur: muscle fibers become tougher and connective tissue becomes tenderer. The time required to cook a specific cut of meat by any method depends on the composition of the meat, size, weight, and shape of the cut.

Tender cuts of meat, cooked by dry-heat methods (roasting, broiling, grilling, frying) to a relatively low temperature (rare, for example), result in tender juicy products. Less-tender cuts must be cooked for longer periods by moist-heat methods (braising, cooking in liquid) to soften connective tissue, prevent surface drying, and develop flavor. If using a marinade, refrigerate the meat at least six to eight hours in an acidic liquid, such as wine, vinegar, or lemon juice. Timetables are guides to approximate cooking times required for meat cuts to reach the desired internal temperature, or desired tenderness

DRY HEAT METHODS

Roasting — this cooking method is recommended for larger cuts of beef, veal, lamb, and pork. Season meat with herbs, spices, or other seasoning before, during, or after roasting. Place meat fat side up on a rack in a shallow roasting pan. In some roasts, rib bones serve as a rack. Insert meat thermometer to the center of the largest muscle. Do not add water or cover. Roast in a slow oven, 300 to 325°F (150–160°C), to the desired doneness. No basting is necessary. Remove roast 5°F (3°C) below desired doneness. The temperature of the meat will rise 5°F (3°C) during standing for 15 to 20 minutes, and the roast will be easier to carve and more moist. See Table 4.3.

Oven Broiling — broiling is suitable for tender steaks and chops; kabobs; pork ribs; sliced ham; bacon; butterflied lamb leg; and ground meat patties or meatballs. Steaks and chops should be at least ¾ inch (2 cm) thick, and ham should be at least ½ inch (1 cm) thick. Less tender cuts, such as beef flank or top round steak, and veal, lamb, and pork shoulder chops, also may be broiled, if they have been marinated. Trim the outer edge of fat. Place thinner cuts of meat (¾ inch to 1 inch or 2 to 2.5 cm thick) on rack of broiler pan 2 to 3 inches (5–7.5 cm) from heat. Allow 3 to 6 inches (7.5–15 cm) for thicker cuts. Broil until the top side is brown, then turn and brown the other side. To test steaks or chops for doneness, cut a small slit in the center away from the bone and check the color of the meat. Season, if desired.

Grilling (Barbecuing) — grilling is actually a method of broiling. Meat can be grilled on a grid or rack over coals or heated ceramic briquettes. Although usually done outdoors, grilling can be done in the kitchen with special types of range tops or small appliances. Start the fire as the manufacturer's instructions indicate. Spread coals in a single layer after they reach the gray ash stage. Low to medium cooking temperatures should be used. To lower the temperature, spread coals farther apart or raise the grid. To make the fire hotter, move the coals closer together and tap off ash. The temperature of the coals can be checked by cautiously holding a hand 4 inches (10 cm) above the coals. Count the number of seconds before the heat forces the removal of the hand. Check the following chart.

CHARCOAL TEMPERATURE FOR GRILLING

Time	Temperature
2 seconds	Hot (high)
3 seconds	Medium-hot
4 seconds	Medium*
5 seconds	Low*
6 to 7 seconds	Very low

* Recommended cooking temperature for meat

For direct cooking, arrange coals in a single layer directly under the food. Use this method for steaks, ham slices, chops, kabobs, and other quickly cooked foods. For larger roasts and steaks, which require longer cooking at lower temperatures, use indirect cooking. This method cooks food by reflecting heat, similar to the way in which a conventional oven cooks. Arrange an equal number of briquettes on each side of the grate, ignite, and make sure the coals are burning equally on both sides. If necessary, move the coals from one side to the other. Place an aluminum foil drip pan between the coals. Arrange the meat on the grid above the drip pan. Cover with damper open and cook as the recipe directs.

Turning the meat during indirect cooking is not necessary. Baste meat with marinade or sauce throughout cooking time, if desired. If the basting sauce contains a large amount of sugar or other ingredients that burn easily, limit basting to the last 15 to 20 minutes. Cooking time can be affected by the type of equipment used, the cooking temperature maintained, the weather, wind velocity, and desired doneness. Discard any marinade not cooked with the meat.

PAN-BROILING

Pan-broiling is a faster, more convenient method than oven broiling for cooking thinner steaks and chops and bacon. Place the meat in a preheated, heavy frying pan, or on a griddle. Most meat cuts have enough fat to prevent sticking; however, the cooking surface may be lightly brushed or sprayed with oil when pan-broiling very lean cuts. No oil is needed with a nonstick frying pan. Do not add water or cover. For cuts thicker than ¼ inch (0.6 cm), cook at medium heat, turning occasionally. Cuts less than ¼ inch (0.6 cm) thick should be cooked at medium-high. Turn more than once to ensure even cooking. Remove fat as it accumulates so that meat does not fry. Cook until brown on both sides. Do not overcook. To test doneness, cut a small slit in the center or close to the bone and check the color of the meat.

Pan-frying — in pan-frying, a small amount of fat is added to the frying pan and fat is allowed to accumulate during cooking. This method is suitable for small or thin cuts of lean meat; thin strips; and pounded, scored, or other tenderized cuts that do not need prolonged heating for tenderization. Brown meat on both sides in small amount of oil. Some cuts will cook in the fat that comes from the meat. Lean cuts, such as cubed steak or cuts, which are floured or breaded, require additional oil on the surface of the pan to prevent sticking. If there is a coating, seasonings may be added to the coating ingredients. Otherwise, the meat may be seasoned after browning. Do not cover the meat or the meat will lose its crisp texture. Cook at medium heat, turning occasionally to promote uniform cooking.

Stir-frying — stir-frying is similar to pan-frying except the food is stirred almost continuously. Cooking is done with high heat, using small or thin pieces of meat. Partially freeze meat to facilitate slicing. Slice meat across the grain into thin, uniform slices, strips, or pieces. If desired, marinate while other ingredients are prepared. Cook meat and vegetables separately and then combine. Place meat in a small amount of hot oil in wok or large frying pan. Stir-fry about a half-pound (0.2 kg) at a time. Cook at a high temperature, sliding the spatula under the meat and turning continuously with a scooping motion.

TABLE 4.3
ROASTING TIMETABLE FOR MEAT

| Cut | Weight | | Oven Temperature | | Approximate Cooking Time (Minutes per Pound) | | |
---	Pounds	Kilo-grams	°F	°C	Rare	Medium	Well Done
Beef							
Rib Roast	4 to 6	2 to 3	300 – 325	150 – 160	26 to 32	27 to 30	40 to 42
	6 to 8	3 to 3.6	300 – 325	150 – 160	23 to 25	34 to 38	32 to 35
Rib Eye Roast	4 to 6	2 to 3	350	180	18 to 20	20 to 22	22 to 24
Boneless Rump Roast	4 to 6	2 to 3	300 – 325	150 – 160		25 to 27	28 to 30
Round Tip Roast	3.5 to 4	1.6 to 2	300 – 325	150 – 160	30 to 35	35 to 38	38 to 40
	6 to 8	3 to 4	300 – 325	150 – 160	22 to 25	25 to 30	30 to 35
Top Round Roast	4 to 6	2 to 3	300 – 325	150 – 160	20 to 25	25 to 28	28 to 30
Tenderloin Roast - Half	2 to 3	1 to 1.5	425	220		35 to 45 total time	
Tenderloin Roast - Whole	4 to 6	2 to 3	425	220		35 to 45 total time	
Ground Beef Loaf (9"x 5"; 3.6 x 2cm)	1.5 to 2.5	0.7 to 1	300 – 325	150 –160		60 to 90 total time	
Veal							
Loin Roast Boneless	2 to 3	1 to 1.5	300 – 325	150 – 160		18 to 20	22 to 24
Loin Roast Bone-In	3 to 4	1.5 to 2	300 – 325	150 – 160		34 to 36	38 to 40
Rib Roast	4 to 5	2 to 2.3	300 – 325	150 – 160		25 to 27	29 to 31
Crown Roast 12-14 ribs	7.5 to 9.5	3.4 to 4.3	300 – 325	150 – 160		19 to 21	21 to 23
Rib Eye Roast	2 to 3		300 – 325	150 – 160		26 to 28	30 to 33
Rump Roast Boneless	2 to 3		300 – 325	150 – 160		33 to 35	37 to 40
Shoulder Roast Boneless	2.5 to 3		300 – 325	150 – 160		31 to 34	34 to 37

ROASTING TIMETABLE FOR MEAT (CONTINUED)

Cut	Weight		Oven Temperature		Approximate Cooking Time (Minutes per Pound)		
	Pounds	Kilo-grams	°F	°C	Rare	Medium	Well Done
Pork							
Loin Roast Center-Bone-In	3 to 5	1.5 to 2.3	325	160		20 to 25	26 to 31
Top Loin Double	3 to 4	1.5 to 2	325	160		29 to 34	33 to 38
Top Loin Single	2 to 4	1 to 2	325	160		23 to 33	30 to 40
Crown Roast	6 to 10	3 to 4.5	325	160			20 to 25
Tenderloin Roast Whole	0.5 to 1	0.2 to 0.5	425	220		27 to 29 total time	30 to 32 total time
Ribs-Backribs			325	160	Cook until tender – 90 to 105 total time		
Pork Smoked (Fully cooked)							
Whole-Boneless*	8 to 12	4 to 5	300 – 325	150 – 160	140	60	13 to 17
Whole-Bone-In**	14 to 16	6 to 7	300 – 325	150 – 160	140	60	12 to 14
Half-Boneless*	6 to 8	3 to 3.6	300 – 325	150 – 160	140	60	17 to 20
Half-Bone-In**	6 to 8	3 to 3.6	300 – 325	150 – 160	140	60	14 to 17
Portion-Boneless	3 to 4	1.5 to 2	300 – 325	150 – 160	140	60	20 to 23
Pork							
Canadian Style Bacon (Fully cooked)	2 to 4	1 to 2	300 – 350	150 – 180	140	60	20 to 30
Lamb							
Leg Roast Whole Bone-In	7 to 9	3 to 4	325	160	15 to 20	20 to 25	25 to 30
Leg Roast Whole Boneless	4 to 7	2 to 3	325	160	25 to 30	30 to 35	35 to 40
Shank-Half	3 to 4	1.5 to 2	325	160	30 to 35	40 to 45	45 to 50
Sirloin-Half	3 to 4	1.5 to 2	325	160	25 to 30	35 to 40	45 to 50
Shoulder Roast Boneless	3.5 to 5	1.6 to 2.3	325	160	30 to 35	35 to 40	40 to 45

NOTES: Cooking times are based on meat taken directly from the refrigerator.
Smaller roasts require more minutes per pound than larger roasts.
Cooking times are approximate.
* Add ½ cup (125 ml) water, cover tightly, and cook as directed.
** Cover tightly and cook as directed.

MOIST HEAT METHODS

Braising — in some areas of the country, "fricassee" and "braising" are interchangeable terms. Two popular examples of braised meats are pot roast and Swiss steak. To braise, first dredge the meat with flour or coat with crumbs, if desired. Then, slowly brown the meat on all sides in a heavy pan in just enough oil to prevent sticking; drain the drippings; and season the meat with salt, herbs, and spices. Browning develops flavor and color. Cuts with sufficient fat do not require additional fat, unless they have been coated with flour or crumbs. Next, add a small amount of liquid (2 Tbsp to ½ cup; 30–125 ml) such as water, tomato juice, wine, and meat or vegetable stock. Cover tightly and simmer on low heat on top of the range or in a 300°F (150–160°C) oven until meat is fork-tender. Check occasionally to make sure liquid does not dry out; add more if necessary. Sauce or gravy may be made from liquid in the pan. Braising times for various cuts of meat are:

Round Steak (¾" to 1", 2–2.5 cm)	1 to 1½ hours
Beef Chuck and Pot Roasts	1¾ to 3 hours
Short Ribs	1½ to 2½ hours
Beef Cubes (1½," 3.7 cm)	1½ to 2½ hours
Veal Shoulder Roast	2 to 2½ hours
Spareribs and Backribs	1½ hours
Pork Cubes (1" to 1¼"; 2.5–to 3 cm)	45 to 60 minutes
Lamb Breast	1½ to 2 hours
Lamb Shanks	1 to 1½ hours

In general, the longer the meat is braised, the tenderer it will be. Meat also can be braised in cooking bags designed specifically for oven use. The benefit is a reduction in cooking time for larger cuts of meat. No additional liquid is needed because moisture is drawn from the meat as it cooks. Follow manufacturer's instructions for best results.

Cooking in liquid — less tender cuts of meat can be covered with liquid and gently simmered until tender. The temperature of the liquid should not rise about 195°F (90°C) because boiling (212°F or 100°C) toughens meat protein. The three ways to cook in liquid are simmering, stewing, and poaching. Simmering (for large cuts) and stewing (for small pieces) are used for less tender cuts of meats. To simmer or stew, brown meat on all sides in a large, heavy pan or Dutch oven; drain drippings. Corned beef and cured and smoked pork need not be browned. Completely cover the meat with water or stock and season as desired. Cover tightly and simmer (do not boil) until meat is fork-tender. When vegetables are to be cooked with the meat, add them whole or in pieces near end of cooking period. When done, remove meat and vegetables to a platter or casserole and keep hot. The cooking liquid may be reduced or thickened for a sauce or gravy. Approximate cooking times are:

Beef for Stew (1" to 2"; 2.5–5 cm)	2 to 3 hours
Fresh or Corned Beef Brisket (2½ to 3½ lb; 1–1.5 kg)	2½ to 3½ hours
Beef Shank Cross Cuts (1" to 1½"; 2.5–3.7 cm)	2½ to 3½ hours
Boneless Breast of Veal	1 to 1½ hours
Lamb and Pork for Stew (1 to 1½ lb; 0.5–0.7 kg)	1½ to 2 hours
Country Style Pork Ribs	2 to 2½ hours

Sous Vide — this method of moist heat cooking involves sealing meat in a packet and cooking it at a precise and constant temperature in a water bath. The result is tender and juicy meat that may be later seared for increased visual and flavor enhancement.

INTERNAL TEMPERATURE

The degree of doneness for meat can be accurately determined by measuring internal temperature with a standard meat thermometer. The thermometer should be inserted into the roast surface at a slight angle or through the end of the roast so the tip of the thermometer is in the thickest portion of the cut, but is not resting in fat or against the bone. Following are internal temperatures for preparing meat:

Beef and Lamb		
Rare	140°F	60°C
Medium rare	150°F	65°C
Medium	160°F	70°C
Well done	170°F	80°C
Veal		
Medium	160°F	70°C
Well done	170°F	80°C
Pork (fresh and cured)		
Medium	160°F	70°C
Well done	170°F	80°C
Ham		
Fully cooked	140°F	60°C

COOKING FROZEN MEATS

Frozen meat may be defrosted in the refrigerator in the original wrapper and cooked according to directions for meat that has not been frozen, or it may be unwrapped and cooked in the frozen state. Additional cooking time is needed when cooking frozen meat. Frozen roasts require 30 to 50 percent more cooking time than roasts started at refrigerator temperature. The additional time needed for cooking steaks and chops varies according to surface area and thickness of the meat and the cooking temperature. Thick frozen steaks, chops, and meat patties must be broiled farther from the heat than those that have been defrosted. This allows the internal temperature to reach the desired level without excessive surface browning. When pan-broiling frozen steaks or chops, a heated frying pan should be used for defrosting the surface rapidly and browning on all sides. The heat should be reduced after browning and the meat turned often so it will cook evenly.

COOKING VARIETY MEATS

All variety meats may be simmered or braised. Some, such as calves liver and lamb or veal kidneys, may be broiled. Regardless of the method, variety meats are usually cooked until well done.

MICROWAVES AND FOOD SYSTEMS

MEAT

The best cuts of meat for microwave cooking are tender, high quality, boneless, and uniform in shape. Bone tends to cause uneven cooking due to the reflective effect on microwaves. Popular meat choices are ground beef; steaks; chops; small roasts; country style ribs or spareribs; bacon and other smoked and cured meat; and precooked, skinless sausage.

As a general rule when microwaving meat dishes, use medium (50 percent) power or medium-low (30 percent) power to ensure tender, flavorful, and evenly cooked meat. Following are some additional tips for promoting even cooking:

- Cut meat into uniform pieces or form ground meat into donut-shaped patties, ½ (1.2 cm) thick.

- Arrange uniform meat shapes, such as meatballs, in a circle on microwave safe dish, leaving center empty. For chops, place meatier portion to outside of dish, with the bone toward the center.

- Stir meat strips several times during cooking, moving the less cooked pieces to the outside and the more cooked pieces to the inside.

- Stir soups, stews, and other dishes with high liquid content several times to distribute the heat.

- Turn meat over several times or rotate dish ¼ to ½ turn at intervals.

- Meat dishes should be covered with a lid or heavy-duty plastic wrap, turned back at one corner. The steam created will help food cook more evenly. Be sure plastic wrap does not touch the food.

A standing period of 10 to 20 minutes may be needed for heat to penetrate the center of the meat after microwaving. When estimating cooking time, allow for a rise in internal temperature of 5 to 10°F (3–6°C) during standing. The slower the cooking and the smaller the mass, the shorter the standing time required. The following internal temperatures are suggested as a guide for determining microwave cooking:

Beef		
Rare	130 to 135°F	55 to 57°C
Medium	150 to 155°F	66 to 69°C
Well done	160 to 165°F	71 to 74°C
Lamb		
Medium	150 to 155°F	66 to 69°C
Well done	160 to 165°F	71 to 74°C
Pork (fresh and cured)		
Well done	160 to 165°F	71 to 74°C
Ham (fully cooked)	130 to 135°F	55 to 57°C

CHAPTER 5: Fish and Shellfish

NUTRITIVE VALUE

The consumption of fish (finfish and shellfish) has risen dramatically within the last decade, primarily because consumers are increasingly aware that fish is one of the most nutritious foods.

PROTEIN CONTENT

Fish contains a complete protein with little connective tissue and is easily cooked until tender. Most species have 17 to 23 percent protein.

VITAMIN AND MINERAL CONTENT

Fishery products are a good source of many vitamins, especially niacin, B6 and B12. Fish, particularly shellfish, is known for its mineral content, with certain species having substantial amounts of calcium, iron, copper, chromium, and/or zinc and other trace minerals. The flesh of both saltwater and freshwater fish is quite low in sodium content, with finfish averaging about 50 mg of sodium in a 3.5 ounce (100 g) raw portion. Shellfish are higher in sodium. Shrimp and oysters contain 235 and 250 mg of sodium per 3.5 ounces (100 g), respectively. Pickled, canned, and smoked fish and surimi seafood have added sodium.

FAT CONTENT

The fat content of fish can range from as low as 1.6 g in ocean perch to 8.6 g in salmon per 3.5 ounces (100 g) portion of uncooked seafood and averages about two grams of fat and 85 kilocalories per 3.5 ounces (100 g).

The lipid in fish is high in polyunsaturated fat. Many fish contain omega-3 fatty acids, which are particularly nutritious forms of fat. The cholesterol content of a 3.5 ounce (100 g) portion of finfish averages about 60 mg, similar to amounts found in pork, beef, and the dark meat of chicken. Most shellfish have moderate levels of cholesterol, ranging from 35 to 90 mg per 3.5 ounce (100 g) portion. Shrimp and squid are higher in cholesterol (about 150 and 200 mg, respectively) but, like all fish, both are low in total fat and saturated fat. Fish is classified as either "lower fat" or "higher fat," which affects the preferred cooking method. Species with less than 5 percent fat content are considered "lean" and are usually characterized by a mild flavor and lighter colored flesh. Species that have a fat content of 5 percent or higher are considered "fat," with a more distinctive flavor and a darker color to the flesh.

MARKET FORMS

There are over 500 species of fish and shellfish commercially available in the United States today. They are marketed fresh, frozen, canned, dried, salted, smoked, and in many convenience forms.

Fresh and frozen fish are marketed in various forms. The following are the most common:

Whole or round fish are sold just as they came from the water. Before cooking, they must be eviscerated.

Drawn fish have been eviscerated and, usually, scaled.

Dressed fish have been scaled and eviscerated and the head, tail, and fins have been removed. A small dressed fish is called pan-dressed.

Fillets are the sides of a fish cut away from the backbone. They may be purchased with the skin on or off and may have small rib or pin bones.

Butterfly or kited fillets are both sides of a fish cut away from the backbone and left connected by the uncut flesh and skin of the back or belly.

Steaks are cross sections of a large dressed fish, typically ¾ to 1 inch (2 to 3 cm) thick. Usually, the skin is left on and a cross-section of the backbone remains. In the case of very large fish (such as some tuna), the fish is cut into loins before steaking and therefore has neither skin nor bone.

Chunks are cross-section portions of large dressed fish, having a cross-section of backbone as the only bone. They are cut much like a beef or pork roast and are ready to cook as purchased.

Raw breaded fish portions are cut from frozen fish blocks coated with a batter, breaded, packaged, and frozen. They are ready to cook as purchased.

Fried fish portions and **fried fish sticks** are cut from frozen fish blocks, coated with a batter, breaded, fully or partially cooked, packaged, and frozen. They are ready to heat and serve as purchased.

Canned fish have been dressed or filleted, mechanically sized and placed into a can that is then sealed and heated. Many species of fish are available canned. Among them are salmon, tuna, sardines, mackerel, shrimp, oysters, and clams. They may be served as purchased.

Salmon, canned on the Pacific Coast, is usually sold by the name of the species. These differ in fat content, color, texture, and flavor. The higher priced varieties are deeper red in color and have a higher oil content than the less costly ones (in descending order: sockeye, chinook or king, coho or silver, and chum or keta).

Tuna canned in the United States is produced from several species of tuna. Albacore, a very light meat, is the only tuna to be labeled white-meat tuna. The other species (yellowfin, blackfin, bluefin, and skipjack) are labeled light-meat tuna. Fancy or solid pack tuna usually contains three or four large pieces packed in oil or water. Chunk, flaked, and grated-style packs contain mechanically sized pieces packed in oil or water.

Sardines are small, immature sea herrings that are packed in water, oil, mustard, or tomato sauce.

Cured fish are either salted or smoked and include salt herring, salmon, salmon eggs, chubs, sablefish, sturgeon, whitefish, mackerel, and mullet. Lox is a mildly cured salmon.

Surimi seafood is an imitation shellfish product made from a mild-flavored finfish, usually Alaskan pollock. The freshly caught fish is made into a paste and then formed into the shape, texture, and color of a shellfish, most commonly crab meat. The processing involves the addition of certain stabilizers, binders, and flavorings, often including real shellfish or a shellfish extract. Surimi seafood is pre-cooked and may or may not be breaded. The nutrient value of unbreaded surimi seafood is similar to that of finfish but has a higher sodium content. It is generally lower in cost than the shellfish it imitates.

Market forms of shellfish are:

Shucked — removed from its shell

Green, headless — usually refers to raw, unprocessed shrimp

Peeled and deveined (P&D) — means shrimp without its shell or black vein

Live — means in shell and alive

IQF — individually quick frozen

SIGNS OF FRESHNESS

FRESH FINFISH

Good quality fresh (unfrozen) finfish have the following characteristics:

- The flesh is firm, not separating or soft. It springs back when pressed gently.

- The odor is fresh and mild. Do a "nasal appraisal" before purchasing.

- The eyes are bright, clear, and often protruding. As the fish loses freshness, the eyes become cloudy, pink, and sunken.

- The gills are bright red or pink and are free from slime.

Avoid fish with dull colored gills that are gray, brown, or green.

- The skin is shiny, with scales that adhere tightly. Characteristic colors and markings may begin to fade soon after the fish is removed from the water.

- The intestinal cavity is clean and pink.

FRESH SHELLFISH

Different species of shellfish vary greatly in terms of market forms and physical characteristics. Look for the following signs of freshness when buying fresh (unfrozen) shellfish:

- The odor is fresh and mild.

- The flesh of shrimp and spiny (southern) lobster is firm. The shell is free of black spots, called melanosis, which are a sign of aging.

- Oysters, clams, and muscles in the shell are alive, as indicated by a tightly closed shell or one that closes upon handling. If a shell opens slightly, tap it with a knife, and it will close. Discard any that do not.

- Uncooked crabs and northern lobsters are alive, as indicated by leg movement. They will not be very active if they have been refrigerated, but they should move a least a little. Also, the tail of a live lobster curls under tightly when it is handled. Discard any uncooked crabs and northern lobsters that do not show these signs of life.

- Fresh shucked oysters are in a clear, slightly milky, or light gray liquid called liquor. Oysters are usually creamy white but there are color variations depending on variety and diet.

- The smaller bay and calico scallops are usually creamy white, though there may be some normal light tan or pink coloration. The larger sea scallops are generally creamy white, though they may show some normal light orange or pink color.

- Crab meat has a fresh, mild odor.

FROZEN FISH

Fishery products that are sold in the frozen form are usually packed during the seasons of abundance, at the peak of freshness, and are held in cold storage until ready for distribution. Thus, the consumer is given the opportunity to select varied species of fish throughout the year and at better prices. High quality frozen fish that are properly processed, packaged, and held will remain in good condition for relatively long periods of time.

Frozen fish of good quality have the following characteristics:

- The fish is solidly frozen when purchased.

- The flesh has no discoloration or freezer burn (a dry, white, or grayish "cottony" appearance.

- The fish has little or no odor. When thawed, it has a mild odor.

- The wrapping is intact and is of moisture/vapor-proof material.

- There is little or no air space between the fish and the wrapping, and there are no ice crystals or frost in the package, which indicates that a variation in temperature has occurred.

HOW MUCH TO BUY

The amount of fish to buy per serving varies with the market form, the recipe to be used, and the yield of edible flesh for the species. Consider about 3 ounces (85 g) of cooked, edible flesh as a serving. The following list can help to determine how much fish to buy per serving.

Finfish	
Whole	¾ pound (350 g)
Dressed, pan-dressed	½ pound (250 g)
Fillet, steaks	⅓ pound (140 g)
Portions	⅓ pound (140 g)
Sticks	¼ pound (125 g)
Canned	⅙ pound (75 g)
Shellfish	
Crab, cooked meat	¼ pound (125 g)
Crabs, live	1 to 2 pounds (500 g to 1 kg)

Shellfish	
Lobster, cooked meat	⅓ pound (140 g)
Lobster, whole	1 to 2 pounds (500 g to 1 kg)
Mussels, live	12
Oysters, clams, live	6
Oysters, clams, shucked	¼ pint (125 ml)
Oysters, clams, breaded	4 to 6
Scallops, shucked	¼ pound (125 g)
Shrimp, unpeeled, headless	½ pound (250 g)
Shrimp, cooked, peeled	¼ pound (125 g)
Shrimp, breaded	4 to 6
Squid, whole	½ pound (250 g)
Squid, cleaned	¼ pound (125 g)

STORING AND THAWING

Fresh fishery products that are to be cooked the day of purchase should be stored immediately in the coldest part of the refrigerator in the original wrapper. Fish that is to be held for up to two days before cooking should be rinsed, patted dry, rewrapped in clean wrapping, and placed on a bed of ice to prevent dehydration before refrigerating. For optimal quality, do not hold fresh fish in the refrigerator longer than two days before cooking. A storage temperature of 32 to 40°F (4°C) is needed to maintain the quality of the product.

Fish that is purchased fresh may be successfully frozen at home. There are a number of ways to properly freeze fish, but the primary concern with all methods is to keep air away from the product. It should be wrapped in a moisture/vapor-proof wrapping (paper, plastic, and/or foil) or frozen in water. Frozen fishery products should be placed in the freezer in their original moisture/vapor-proof wrapping immediately after purchase, unless the fish is to be thawed for cooking. A storage temperature of 0°F (-18°C) or lower is necessary to maintain quality. At higher temperatures, chemical changes cause fish to lose color, flavor, texture, and nutritive value. Generally, higher fat species may be held in the freezer up to four months without significant loss of quality, and lean species may be frozen for up to one year. It is, however, best to use frozen products soon after purchase for optimal quality.

When thawing fish, consider the following:

- Schedule thawing so that the fish will be cooked soon after it is thawed. Do not hold thawed fish longer than a day before cooking.

- Place frozen packages in the refrigerator to thaw, allowing 18 to 24 hours or longer for thawing a one-pound (500 g) package.

- If quicker thawing of an unbreaded product is necessary, place the frozen package under cold running water or in cold water to thaw. Allow ½ to 1 hour per pound (500 g) of frozen product.

- Thaw fish in the microwave on the defrost setting for four to five minutes per pound (500 g), just until it is pliable enough to handle.

- Do not thaw fish at room temperature or in warm water.

- Avoid refreezing fish, as it results in a lower quality product with a higher bacteria count.

- For prepared products, including fish sticks and portions, follow the manufacturer's instructions.

- Frozen fillets and steaks may be cooked without thawing if additional cooking time is allowed.

SAFE HANDLING

All raw foods, including finfish and shellfish, contain bacteria. Fish should be handled as any perishable food product: keep it properly refrigerated, cook it adequately, and handle it with safety in mind.

To maintain wholesomeness and quality, always follow these guidelines:

- Know the fish retailer. Buy fishery products from approved, licensed stores and markets.

- Purchase raw shellfish carefully. Buy raw oysters, clams, and mussels only from approved, licensed, reputable sources. If in doubt, ask to see the certified shipper's tag that accompanies all live mollusks; look for a shipper number on containers of shucked oysters.

- Keep fish cold.

- Refrigerate live shellfish properly. Live oysters, clams, and mussels should be stored under well-ventilated refrigeration, not in airtight plastic bags or storage containers. Burlap, net or heavy paper bags work well, as do plastic bags that are left open. Live lobsters and crabs should be stored similarly, with a covering of damp paper towels.

- Keep live shellfish alive until cooking. Discard any that have died during storage.

- Do not cross-contaminate. Handle and store raw and cooked products separately. Once a cutting board, colander, or platter has been in contact with raw finfish or shellfish, wash it thoroughly before using it for cooked products.

- Cook fish and shellfish thoroughly (145°F [63°C]).

- Harvest fish carefully. If fish or shellfish are caught from local waters, make sure the waters are approved for harvest. Always carry plenty of ice and do not catch more than can be chilled immediately.

EATING RAW FISH AND SHELLFISH

Many consumers enjoy raw fish. Just as the consumption of raw or undercooked beef, pork, chicken, and eggs carries a degree of risk for foodborne gastrointestinal illness, so does the consumption of undercooked fish, raw fish (i.e., sashimi, sushi, ceviche), and raw oysters, clams, and mussels. Here are some tips to reduce the risk:

- Buy only the highest quality fish and shellfish; keep it properly refrigerated and use it the same day of purchase.

- If not previously frozen, hard freeze fish intended for preparation of sashimi, sushi, or ceviche for seven days to avoid the slight risk associated with parasites.

- Be certain that oysters, clams, and mussels come from certified growing waters. Make certain they are kept well refrigerated.

- Never eat raw or undercooked fishery products if seriously ill with a disease that compromises the immune system, such as cancer, HIV/AIDS, alcoholism, liver disease, or kidney disease.

COOKING METHODS

Fish is delicious if properly cooked. Cooking fish develops its flavor, softens the small amount of connective tissue present, and gives the desired texture. Over-cooking fish toughens it, dries it out, destroys the fine flavor, and reduces the yield.

Raw fish has a watery, translucent look. During the cooking process, the moisture in fish becomes milky colored giving the flesh an opaque, whitish tint. When this occurs at the center part of the fish, the fish is properly cooked.

To estimate how long to cook a fish, use the "10-minute rule" as a guideline unless the fish is to be microwaved or deep-fried. Follow these steps:

1. Measure the fish at its thickest point. If other ingredients are added, include them in the measurement.

2. Plan to cook the fish for approximately 10 minutes per inch (2.5 cm) of thickness.

3. Before the estimated cooking time is complete, use a fork or knife, check the fish for doneness at the thickest point. Remove the fish from the heat when finfish are flaky and shellfish are tender; both should no longer be translucent in the center. An internal temperature of 145°F (60°C) ensures the fish is safe to eat. The cooking time required will vary somewhat according to the temperature and cooking method used. Check for doneness early and often.

4. Double the estimated cooking for frozen fish that has not been thawed.

Most fish are quite delicate and tend to break up easily, so handle as little and as gently as possible during and after cooking to preserve appearance.

When choosing a cooking method and recipe for fish, carefully consider the species to be used. Fat fish are usually distinctive in flavor and can therefore be used in recipes with other robust flavors; the higher fat content also helps maintain moisture in the cooked product. Lean species of fish and shellfish should be used with ingredients that will not overpower their milder flavors, and care should be taken to prevent the product from drying out.

One may substitute a different species for the one specified in a recipe as long as it has similar characteristics. Consider the texture, flavor, and fat content.

DRY HEAT METHODS

Baking
Whole fish lend themselves well to baking, as do fillets and steaks. Cut fish into serving-size portions. Arrange on a well-oiled baking dish, and baste with melted butter or margarine, oil, or a marinade. If desired, sprinkle with herbs or spices, citrus juice, or wine. Bake at 375°F (190°C). Turning is not necessary.

Broiling
Choose pan-dressed fish, fillets, steaks, or shellfish for broiling. Prepare the fish as for baking. Place under the broiler, about 3 or 4 inches (8 to 10 cm) from the source of heat. Place thicker cuts of fish farther from the heat than thin ones. Baste frequently; turn halfway through cooking time unless fish is very thin.

Charcoal Broiling/Grilling
Fillets, steaks, and shellfish are good choices for this cooking method. Before heating the grill, lightly brush the grill and the fish with oil. For fish that is 1 inch (3 cm) thick or less, place the grill 2 to 4 inches (5 to 10 cm) away from the coals; for thicker pieces, 5 to 6 inches (12 to 15 cm) away. For particularly delicate fish, use a hinged, wire fish or hamburger basket (oiled); wooden or metal skewers may be used for shrimp or scallops. Turn the fish halfway through the estimated cooking time, basting frequently with oil or sauce.

Deep Fat Frying
Choose fillets, shucked shellfish, and small dressed fish for this method. In a deep-fat fryer, heat enough vegetable oil to float the fish but do not fill the fryer more than half full. Heat the oil to 375°F (190°C). Cut the fish into serving-size portions. Dip the fish into seasoned milk or beaten egg and then into seasoned crumbs, cornmeal, or flour. Or coat with flour and then dip into a batter. Arrange in a fryer basket to be lowered into the fryer or drop gently into the oil and fry until golden brown, flaky, and no longer translucent in the center. Drain on absorbent paper.

Pan-Frying
Pan-frying is an excellent way to cook pan-dressed fish, fillets, and steaks. Prepare the fish as for deep-fat frying. Heat ¼ to ½ inch (6 mm to 1 cm) oil or other fat in a heavy fry pan. Place one layer of fish in the hot fat, taking care not to overload the pan and thus cool the fat. Fry until golden brown on one side, then turn and brown on the other side. Drain on absorbent paper.

Oven-Frying
Fillets are the preferred market form to use for oven-frying. Cut the fish into serving-size portions. Dip the pieces in seasoned milk or other liquid and coat with flour or crumbs such as crackers, bread, or a snack food. Place the fish on a shallow, well-oiled baking pan, drizzle lightly with oil and bake at 450°F (240°C). Turning is not necessary.

MOIST HEAT METHODS

Poaching

Any cut of fish may be poached. Often, shellfish is referred to as "boiled," when actually it is prepared by poaching or simmering. Place just enough liquid to cover the finfish into a shallow, wide pan, such as a large fry pan. A Dutch oven or stockpot may be used for shellfish. The liquid may be plain or lightly salted water, water seasoned with herbs and spices, milk, or a mixture of white wine and water. Cover the pan and heat until the liquid simmers. Gently add the fish, cover, and simmer. After the fish is removed, the liquid may then be reduced and thickened to make a sauce for the fish.

Steaming

Choose any market form of fish for steaming. A steam cooker or any deep pot with a tight cover may be used for steaming fish. If a steaming rack or basket is not available, use a plate or cake rack placed atop an inverted cup or bowl to hold the fish above the water. Pour about 2 inches (5 cm) of water into the pot and bring to a boil. The water may be plain or seasoned with herbs, spices, or wine. Place the fish on a lightly oiled rack, basket, or plate over the boiling water. Cover the pot tightly and steam.

MICROWAVE COOKING

Small whole fish, fillets, and steaks are particularly good choices for microwave cookery. To achieve the best results when microwaving fish, special consideration should be given to the quantity and shape of the fish, the size, shape of the dish, and the wattage and power settings of the oven. Because there are no standard power settings among most oven brands, the cooking time suggested in recipes should be considered only a guideline. Frequent checking for doneness is required, and notations should be made on actual cooking time for future reference. Use the following techniques when microwaving fish:

- Use a shallow dish to allow the fish maximum exposure to the microwaves. Cover the dish with a paper towel, waxed paper, or plastic wrap (vented).

- Arrange the fillets with the thicker parts toward the outside of the dish. The thinner parts, separated by plastic wrap, may be overlapped in the center.

- Use the high power setting and plan to microwave the fish 3 to 5 minutes per pound (500 g). Rotate the dish halfway through the estimated cooking time; turning the fish is not necessary. Check the fish early and often for doneness. If needed, continue to microwave and check for doneness at 1-minute intervals.

COOKING SHELLFISH

There are special considerations for cooking each species of shellfish, particularly regarding cooking times. Cook shellfish lightly, looking for the following signs of doneness.

- When properly cooked, shrimp turn pink with an opaque rather than translucent center. One pound (500 g) of medium or large shrimp requires only 3 to 5 minutes of cooking when being boiled or steamed.

- Shucked mollusks, such as oysters, clams, and mussels, become plump and opaque when cooked. The edges of oysters start to curl.

- Mollusks in the shell open when they are done. Remove individual pieces from the heat as they open. Discard any that do not open.

- Scallops turn milky white in the center when done. Depending on the size and the cooking method, scallops take from 2 to 5 minutes to cook.

- "Boiled" northern lobster turns bright red. When properly cooked, the center of the meat is no longer translucent. Allow 5 to 6 minutes per pound (500 g) in simmering water.

- Spiny lobster turns bright orange with an opaque rather than translucent center. Cooking time in simmering water varies from 8 to 15 minutes, depending on the size and market form.

AQUACULTURE

Aquaculture is the raising of fish or shellfish in tanks, ponds, waterways, or net pens and is one of the fastest growing sectors of the U. S. agricultural industry.

- Worldwide consumer demand for fish continues to increase, while harvests of wild stocks remain static.

- Cultured fish provides consumers with fresh fish year round.

- The aquaculture industry is developing many species, such as hybrid striped bass and tilapia.

Among the species increasingly cultured are catfish, crawfish, shrimp, salmon, tilapia, oysters, clams, scallops, and lobster.

INSPECTION AND GRADING

By the authority of the federal Food, Drug, and Cosmetic Safety Act, the Food and Drug Administration (FDA) of the U.S. Department of Health and Human Services is primarily responsible for the regulation of fish and seafood. FDA conducts inspections of seafood processing operations and evaluates fish handling procedures within each facility. Inspectors analyze and test the products produced in these plants for filth, decomposition, and contaminants. Imported seafood also is overseen by the FDA, which is responsible for wharf examination and product testing.

The National Marine Fisheries Service of the U.S. Department of Commerce (USDC), the Environmental Protection Agency, and coastal state governments all participate in seafood regulation programs that collectively and comprehensively monitor seafood safety.

Inspection and grading of fish and fishery products are voluntary services that the U.S. Department of Commerce makes available to the seafood industry on a fee-for-service basis. Labels of inspected and/or graded fishery products that meet federal standards then may carry U.S. grade and inspection marks with a grade of the product and a statement that the product was packed under federal inspection.

Quality grades include Grade A fishery products, which are top or best quality, uniform in size, practically free from blemishes or defects, and of good flavor; Grade B, which is good quality but not as uniform in size or free from blemishes and defects as the top grade; and Grade C, which is fairly good quality, is considered wholesome and nutritious but may not be as attractive in appearance as the other grades.

The USDC has issued standards for many frozen precooked and raw breaded fishery products to establish minimum percentages of flesh content. The following table (Table 5.1) lists the minimum percent flesh for breaded fishery products bearing the USDC Grade A inspection marks.

TABLE 5.1
MINIMUM FLESH CONTENT REQUIREMENTS FOR USDC-INSPECTED PRODUCTS

Product	USDC Grade Marks (Minimum % of Flesh by Weight)	PUFI Mark[1] (Minimum % of Flesh by Weight)
Fish		
Raw Breaded Fillets	-	50[2]
Precooked Breaded Fillets	-	50
Precooked Crispy/Crunchy Fillets	-	50
Precooked Battered Fillets	-	40
Raw Breaded Portions	75	50
Precooked Breaded Portions	65	50
Precooked Breaded Portions	-	40
Raw Breaded Sticks	72	50
Precooked Breaded Sticks	60	50
Precooked Battered Sticks	-	40
Scallops		
Raw Breaded Scallops	50	50
Precooked Breaded Scallops	50	50
Precooked Crispy/Crunchy Scallops	-	50
Precooked Battered Scallops	-	40
Shrimp		
Lightly Breaded Shrimp	65	65[3]
Raw Breaded Shrimp	50	50[3]
Precooked Crispy/Crunchy Shrimp	-	50
Precooked Battered Shrimp	-	40
Precooked Breaded Shrimp	-	No minimum. Encouraged to put percent on label.[4]

MINIMUM FLESH CONTENT REQUIREMENTS FOR USDC-INSPECTED PRODUCTS
(CONTINUED)

Product	USDC Grade Marks (Minimum % of Flesh by Weight)	PUFI Mark[1] (Minimum % of Flesh by Weight)
Oysters		
Raw Breaded Oysters	-	50[5]
Precooked Breaded Oysters	-	50[5]
Precooked Crispy / Crunchy Oysters	-	50[5]
Precooked Battered Oysters	-	40[5]
Miscellaneous		
Fish and Seafood Cakes	-	35
Extruded and Breaded Products	-	35

[1] PUFI: nonstandardized breaded and battered products. (PUFI = Packed Under Federal Inspection)

[2] No USDC grading standard currently exists.

[3] FDA Standard of Identity requires any product to have 50 percent shrimp flesh by weight. If a product is labeled "lightly" breaded it must contain 65 percent shrimp flesh.

[4] Any product with a Standard of Identity that contains less flesh than the standard requires must be labeled imitation.

[5] Flesh content on oyster products can only be determined on an input weight basis during production.

CHAPTER 6: Poultry and Eggs

POULTRY

Poultry is marketed as ready-to-cook raw poultry and ready-to-eat forms. More poultry is sold as parts, often skinless and boneless, and as further processed products than as whole birds. Many further processed food products include poultry meat as a main ingredient. New packaging techniques, such as modified atmosphere packaging, shelf-stable products, and sous vide products (dishes with fresh ingredients that are vacuum-packed, cooked under vacuum, and chilled), have expanded the variety of refrigerated, canned, and frozen items available.

FEDERAL POULTRY PROGRAMS

All poultry slaughtered in the United States is inspected for wholesomeness by the federal government (U. S. Department of Agriculture [USDA]) or by an equivalent state system. Federal inspection is mandatory for slaughtered poultry moving in interstate commerce. Poultry moving in intrastate commerce is subject to state inspection.

Birds are examined inside and out by an official inspector. Poultry also may be graded for quality by an official grader through a voluntary program. Officially inspected and graded poultry is prepared in processing plants that meet USDA sanitary requirements. The inspection mark (a circle stating "Inspected for Wholesomeness by the U.S. Department of Agriculture") and the grade mark (a shield stating USDA Grade A, B, or C) appear on the package label.

Grades for poultry have been established by USDA. Most poultry identified with a grade mark will be Grade A. It will be fully fleshed, meaty, well formed, have a uniform fat covering, a good clean appearance, and be free from defects such as skin cuts and tears, pinfeathers, bruises, and missing or broken bones.

For each kind of poultry, the USDA also has established classes based essentially on the age of the bird. Unless specified, the birds may be of either sex. The age of the bird affects its tenderness and dictates the cooking method to use. Young birds are tender-meated and can be cooked by any method but are best roasted, broiled, or fried. Mature birds are less tender and need to be braised or stewed.

SAFE HANDLING

Poultry, like many other foods, may contain *Salmonella* bacteria, but proper cooking and handling methods can eliminate any threat to health. Thorough washing under cool running water prior to cooking greatly reduces bacterial hazards. Because salmonella are easily destroyed by heat, all poultry should be cooked to the well-done stage, 165°F (74°C). Juices from the cooked meat should be clear, not pink.

Always thaw poultry in the refrigerator or in cold water, not on the counter. Bacteria multiply rapidly at room temperature.

Wash hands, counter tops, and utensils in hot soapy water between each step in poultry preparation. Bacteria present on raw meat or poultry can get into other food if exposed to the same utensils. For instance, do not cut up raw poultry and then use the same knife or cutting board to prepare other foods unless the knife and board have been washed thoroughly. Be sure the platter that carries the cooked meat to the table is not the same platter that carried the raw meat to the grill.

Cooked poultry that is not eaten immediately should be kept either hot, 140°F (60°C) or hotter, or cold, 40°F (4°C) or colder. Thoroughly reheat leftovers before eating. Bring gravies to a rolling boil before serving. If any of these products are reheated, they should reach 165°F (74°C).

Store poultry for picnics or lunches in an insulated container until ready to eat.

Implementation of the Egg Safety Rule (which establishes requirements for control of *Salmonella enteritidis* in eggs from production through distribution) began in July 2010 for large (50,000 layers+) producers; July 2012 for smaller producers.

IN THE REFRIGERATOR

Store chilled raw poultry in its transparent wrap for one or two days in the coldest part of the refrigerator. If wrapped only in market paper, rinse with cold water, place in a plastic bag on a plate and store at the bottom of the refrigerator. Wrap and store giblets separately.

Cool cooked poultry quickly by wrapping loosely and setting it in the coolest part of the refrigerator.

Remove stuffing from cooked stuffed birds and store in a separate covered container in the refrigerator. Refrigerate broth or gravy promptly.

Use cooked poultry within three to four days. Use stuffing, broth, or gravy within one or two days.

IN THE FREEZER

Both uncooked and cooked poultry may be frozen and stored for several months at 0°F (18°C) or colder. If properly packaged, such products can be kept up to one year. (See Table 6.1 for recommended storage times for maximum quality.) Do not stuff uncooked poultry before freezing. Remove stuffing from cooked poultry and freeze meat and stuffing separately.

THAWING

Keep poultry frozen until ready to thaw or cook. Thaw in the refrigerator in original wrapping (see Table 6.2) or in cold water, changing the water every 30 minutes, or in the microwave following manufacturer's directions. It takes 24 hours to thaw a 4 lb chicken in the refrigerator; cut up pieces, 3 to 9 hours. If placed into a plastic bag and immersed in cold water, chicken can thaw in 2 hours. Cook promptly after thawing. Do not thaw poultry at room temperature.

TABLE 6.1
FREEZER STORAGE TIMETABLE

Poultry Form	Months
Uncooked poultry	
Chicken	
Cut-up	9
Giblets	3
Whole	12
Duck, whole	6
Goose, whole	6
Turkey	
Cut-up	6
Whole	12
Cooked poultry (slices or pieces)	
Covered with broth	6
Not covered with broth	1
Cooked poultry dishes	4 to 6
Fried chicken	4
Poultry gravy or broth	2 to 3

TABLE 6.2
THAWING TIMETABLE IN REFRIGERATOR FOR POULTRY

Poultry Type and Size	Time Required
Chickens	
4 pounds (2 kg) or more	1 to 1½ days
Less than 4 pounds (2 kg)	12 to 16 hours
Ducks	
3 to 7 pounds (1 to 3 kg)	1 to 1½ days
Geese	
6 to 12 pounds (3 to 5 kg)	1 to 2 days
Turkeys	
4 to 12 pounds (2 to 5 kg)	1 to 2 days
12 to 20 pounds (5 to 9 kg)	2 to 3 days
20 to 24 pounds (9 to 10 kg)	3 to 4 days
Pieces of large turkey	
(half, quarter, half breast)	1 to 2 days
Cut-up pieces	3 to 9 hours
Boneless roasts	12 to 18 hours

COOKING METHODS

All poultry should be washed in cold water before cooking and cooked to the well-done stage. Juices should run clear. Whole birds or parts may be roasted, fried, braised, or stewed. Always cook chicken to a well-done stage: 180°F (82°C) for a whole bird; 170°F (76°C) for parts with bone in; and 160°F (71°C) for boneless parts.

DRY HEAT METHODS

Roasting

Allowing about 1 cup (250 ml) stuffing per pound (0.5 kg) of bird, stuff poultry lightly just before roasting. Do not stuff the day before.

Roast on rack in uncovered shallow pan. Do not add water.

Do not partly roast poultry one day and complete roasting the next day.

Roast stuffed or unstuffed poultry in preheated 325°F (160°C) oven. Do not cook at low temperatures overnight.

Use a meat thermometer to determine doneness of medium to large birds. Temperature in the inner thigh (not touching the bone) should reach 180° to 185°F (80° to 85°C) or for turkey roasts, 170°F (77°C). Stuffing should reach 165°F (75°C). For approximate total roasting times of various poultry products see Table 6.3.

To roast commercially stuffed poultry, follow directions on the package. Frozen commercially stuffed poultry is ready for the oven and must not be thawed before cooking. Roast chicken at 350°F (177°C) for 30 minutes per pound of product

Broiling

Chicken, small fryer-roaster turkeys, and ducklings can be broiled satisfactorily. Cut into halves, quarters or pieces. Place cut chicken pieces on rack of broiler pan 5 to 6 inches (7.5 to 15 cm) from heat. Broil on one side until browned, turn, and broil until done. Chicken will require 20 to 30 minutes on the first side and 15 to 20 minutes after turning. Turkey and duck pieces are thicker and require longer broiler time. Allow 60 to 75 minutes total.

Outdoor Broiling

Set broiler racks 6 to 8 inches (15 to 20 cm) from the coals. If meat cooks too fast, raise rack or spread coals farther apart. Broil, turning occasionally, about one hour for chicken, longer for turkey.

Rotisserie Cooking

Whole poultry or large pieces can be cooked on rotisserie equipment. Follow manufacturer's directions.

Frying

Young chickens, capons, Rock Cornish game hens, and small turkeys can be fried. Serving size pieces are easiest to handle and may be coated or uncoated.

To avoid excess fat in the diet, it is wise to prepare fried poultry with a minimum of fat. Removing skin before cooking also reduces fat.

To pan-fry, heat enough fat or oil, about 2 or 3 tablespoons (30 to 45 ml), to cover the bottom of a heavy frying pan. Place meatier pieces in the center of pan, smaller pieces at edges. Brown over medium heat on one side, turn, and brown other side. For chicken, continue to cook slowly, uncovered, until tender, 30 to 45 minutes, or cook in 350°F (180°C) oven until done. For turkey, cover tightly after browning and cook slowly 45 to 60 minutes or until done, turning occasionally. Uncover for the last few minutes to re-crisp, if desired.

To oven-fry, place poultry pieces in a well-greased baking pan. Cook, skin side down, in 400°F (200°C) oven for 30 minutes. Turn and cook 20 to 30 minutes longer or until done. Turkey pieces will need a longer cooking time.

Deep-fat frying, although it produces a desirable crisp coating, also results in a cooked product that is very high in fat content. To cook by this method, coat poultry pieces with a thin batter, flour, or crumbs. Use a deep kettle, filled no more than half full with melted fat or oil (deep enough to cover chicken pieces). Heat fat to 365°F (180°C). Check temperature with a deep-fat thermometer. Fry a few pieces at a time for 10 to 15 minutes. Drain on paper towels to remove excess fat.

Smoking

In some areas, smoking is a popular method for cooking turkeys. Smoking may be done in equipment designed for the purpose or in a covered backyard grill, following manufacturer's directions.

Prepare thawed or fresh unstuffed turkey as for roasting. Soaking in a brine solution before cooking lends a characteristic flavor but is not essential.

Allow the bed of coals to become hot. Add water to the drip pan under the turkey. The temperature of the smoker should be kept between 225 and 300°F (107°C and 150°C) throughout the cooking. To maintain this temperature, add coals every one to two hours. Cook until meat thermometer registers 180°F (80°C) in thigh and 170°F (75°C) in the breast meat, and juices run clear. Cooking time will vary depending on outside temperature, wind, and altitude and may take as long as eight hours. Smoking methods also may be used for preparing geese, ducks, and pheasants.

MOIST HEAT METHODS

Braising

Mature, less tender poultry often requires braising (cooking slowly in a tightly covered pan with a small amount of moisture). Braising of young, tender poultry and boneless turkey roasts is faster than roasting. (See Table 6.4 for braising timetable.)

Place whole or cut up poultry on a rack in roaster or heavy pan and cover tightly. Cook in 400°F (200°C) oven until leg joints move easily and flesh on leg is soft and pliable. To brown, uncover for last 30 minutes of cooking of whole large turkeys or a shorter time for smaller sizes of poultry. Poultry also can be braised on top of the range. Use a heavy, covered pan, add ⅓ cup of water, and follow oven directions. Cook slowly over low to medium heat for 1½ to 2½ hours, adding water if necessary.

Simmering or Stewing

Mature chickens or turkeys need to be simmered or stewed to become tender. Simmer or stew poultry in enough water to barely cover. Add vegetables such as onion and celery if desired. Cover pot and cook over low heat until tender when pierced with a fork. Mature chickens require 1½ to 2 hours; young chickens, ¾ to 1 hour; and young large turkeys, 3 to 3½ hours.

To shorten cooking time, cook in a pressure cooker or pressure saucepan, following the manufacturer's directions.

TABLE 6.3

ROASTING TIMES FOR POULTRY

	Purchased Weight[1]		Approximate Total Roasting Time at 325°F (160°C)	
	Pounds	Kilograms	Fresh or thawed poultry 32° to 40°F (4°C) (Hours)	Frozen poultry 0°F (-18°C) or below (Hours)
Chicken				
Whole				
Broiler–Fryer	2¼ – 3¼	1 – 1.5	1¾ – 2½	2 – 3
Roaster	3¼ – 4½	1.5 – 2	2 – 3	2½ – 3½
Capon	5 – 8½	2 – 4	3 – 4	
Rock Cornish game hen	1 – 2	0.5 – 1	1½ – 2	
Pieces	¼ – ¾	0.1 – 0.3	1 – 2½	1 – 2¾
Duck	4 – 6	2 – 3	2½ – 4	3½ – 4½
Geese	6 – 8	3 – 4	3 – 3½	
Turkey				
Whole, unstuffed	6 – 8	3 – 4	3 – 3½	
	8 – 12	4 – 5	3½ – 4½	
	12 – 16	5 – 7	4½ – 5½	5½ – 6½
	16 – 20	7 – 9	5½ – 6½	
	20 – 24	9 – 10	6½ – 7	7 – 8½
Halves, whole breast	5 – 11	2 – 5	3 – 5½	4½ – 6¼
Quarters, thighs, drumsticks	1 – 3	0.5 – 1.5	2 – 3½	2 – 3¾
Boneless roast	3 – 10	1.5 – 5	3 – 4	

[1] Weight of giblets and neck included for whole poultry.

TABLE 6.4
BRAISING TIMETABLE FOR POULTRY

	Ready-to-Cook Weight[1]		Approximate Total Braising Time	
	Pounds	Kilograms	Fresh or thawed poultry 32° to 40°F (4°C) (Hours)	Frozen poultry 0°F (-18°C) or below (Hours)
Chicken				
Whole				
Broiler–Fryer	2¼ – 3¼	1 – 1.5	1½ – 2¼	2 – 2½
Roaster	3¼ – 4½	1.5 – 2	1¾ – 2½	2½ – 3½
Pieces	¼ – ¾	0.1 – 0.3	½ – 1	¾ – 1½
Wings	¼ – less	0.1	1	1¼
Turkey				
Whole	12 – 16	5 – 7	3½ – 5	4½ – 6
	16 – 20	7 – 9	4½ – 6½	5½ – 7½
	20 – 24	9 – 10	6 – 8	7 – 9
Half, breast	5 – 11	2 – 5	2 – 3¼	3 – 4½
Quarters, thighs, drumsticks	1 – 3	0.5 – 1.5	1 – 2	1¼ – 2¼
Wings	¾ – 1¼	0.3 – 0.5	2 – 2½	2 – 2½
Boneless roast	3 – 10	1.5 – 5	1½ – 5	

[1] Weight of giblets and neck included for whole poultry.

EGGS

Eggs, as discussed in this chapter, refer to chicken eggs unless otherwise noted.

Eggs are a nutrient-dense food with a low calorie count. A large egg contains 213 milligrams of cholesterol, but only about 1.5 grams of saturated fat. Egg protein is of exceptionally high quality. The yolk contains almost half of the egg's protein, and, except for magnesium, riboflavin, and niacin, the yolk is higher in nutrients than the egg white. There is no difference in nutrition, taste, or functional properties between brown and white-shelled eggs.

TABLE 6.5
WEIGHT PER DOZEN EGGS

Jumbo	30 oz.	(850 g)
Extra large	27 oz.	(765 g)
Large	24 oz.	(680 g)
Medium	21 oz.	(595 g)
Small	18 oz.	(510 g)
Peewee	15 oz.	(425 g)

SHELL EGGS

Chicken eggs are marketed according to grade and size standards established by the USDA or by equivalent standards set by state departments of agriculture. The USDA shield on the egg carton means that the eggs have been federally inspected. Most state laws require that the grade, size, date of pack and/or expiration date appear on the carton label. Plants not under USDA inspection are governed by laws of their states.

Size and grade are two entirely different factors bearing no relationship to one another. The interior and exterior quality of the egg determine grade at the time the egg is packed.

Grades are AA, A, and B. Most Grade B eggs go to egg breakers for use in egg products. As the egg ages, the white becomes thinner, allowing the egg to spread more when broken out. This characteristic makes the freshest eggs most desirable when appearance is important, as for poaching or frying. Eggs a week or two old are best for hard cooking, because they can be peeled more easily.

Size is classified according to minimum weight per dozen.

Although eggs are sold by number of eggs per carton, it is easier to determine which size is the best to buy by comparing the price per pound, as shown in Table 6.6.

TABLE 6.6
COMPARATIVE PRICES PER DOZEN EGGS

Small (18 oz) (510 g)	Medium (21 oz) (595 g)	Large (24 oz) (680 g)	X-Large (27 oz) (765 g)	Jumbo (30 oz) (850 g)	Price/lb (16 oz) (454 g)
$.60	$.70	$.80	$.89	$.99	$.53
.64	.74	.85	.95	1.06	.56½
.68	.79	.90	1.01	1.13	.60
.71	.83	.95	1.06	1.18	.63
.75	.87	1.00	1.12	1.25	.66½
.79	.92	1.05	1.18	1.31	.70
.82	.96	1.10	1.23	1.37	.73
.86	1.00	1.15	1.29	1.43	.76½
.90	1.05	1.20	1.35	1.50	.80
.93	1.09	1.25	1.40	1.56	.83
.97	1.14	1.30	1.46	1.62	.86½
1.01	1.18	1.35	1.52	1.69	.90
1.05	1.22	1.40	1.57	1.74	.93
1.09	1.27	1.45	1.63	1.81	.96½
1.13	1.31	1.50	1.69	1.88	1.00

SIZE EQUIVALENTS

Any size egg may be used for frying, scrambling, cooking in the shell, or poaching, but recipes are usually based on the use of large eggs. To substitute another size, use Table 6.7.

TABLE 6.7
TO MAKE 1 CUP

Egg Size	Whole	Whites	Yolks
Jumbo	4	5	11
X-Large	4	6	12
Large	5	7	14
Medium	5	8	16
Small	6	9	18

CARE AND HANDLING

Although a small percentage of shell eggs may contain *Salmonella,* eggs are a safe food when handled like other perishable foods. Refrigeration is of prime importance in preserving egg quality and safety.

- Buy eggs at retail from refrigerated cases only. For food service, use only eggs delivered under refrigeration.

- Refrigerate with large end up in cartons or cases, at 40°F (4°C) or colder. Properly refrigerated eggs keep 4 to 5 weeks past the pack date without significant loss of quality.

- Use only clean, uncracked eggs.

- Wash cutting boards and all utensils used in egg preparation before using for other foods.

- Do not leave broken-out eggs or egg dishes at room temperature more than two hours including preparation and service. If not served immediately, keep egg dishes below 40°F (4°C) or above 140°F (60°C).

- To store unbroken yolks, cover with water in a tightly covered container, refrigerate, and use in one or two days, or hard cook them, drain well, and refrigerate in a tightly sealed container up to four or five days.

- Refrigerate raw whites in a tightly covered container for up to four days.

- Refrigerate hard-cooked unpeeled eggs and use within a week.

FREEZING EGGS

Broken-out eggs can be frozen successfully. Label containers with date, number of eggs, and whether salt or sugar have been added.

Whites — pour into freezer containers and seal tightly.

Yolks — the gelation property of frozen yolks makes them almost impossible to use in a recipe unless ⅛ teaspoon salt (0.5 ml) or 1½ teaspoon (7 ml) sugar or corn syrup per ¼ cup (60 ml) or 4 yolks is added before freezing.

Whole eggs — beat just until blended and pour into freezer containers. Salt, sugar, or corn syrup needs to be added because of the presence of the yolks.

TO USE FROZEN EGGS

Thaw under running cold water or overnight in the refrigerator. Use immediately. Whites will beat to a greater volume if allowed to stand at room temperature about 30 minutes.

2 Tbsp (30 ml) thawed egg white = 1 large fresh egg white

1 Tbsp (15 ml) thawed egg yolk = 1 large fresh yolk

3 Tbsp (45 ml) thawed whole egg = 1 large fresh egg

Use thawed frozen eggs only in dishes that are thoroughly cooked.

MICROWAVE COOKING

Because few foods are as heat-sensitive as eggs, a reduced power level of 200 to 300 watts is recommended for all egg dishes except omelets, poached eggs with water added, and scrambled eggs.

Do not cook raw eggs in their shells or reheat peeled or unpeeled hard-cooked eggs. They will explode. Rapid build-up of steam can cause yolks of broken-out eggs to explode. Always prick yolks of unbeaten eggs and cover container with waxed paper or plastic wrap to avoid splattering.

Microwave cooking is not recommended for soufflés and puffy omelets.

For quick, hard-cooked eggs, separate yolks and whites into two small bowls. Stir yolks. Cover and cook separately on reduced power (200 to 300 watts), stirring once or twice. Allow 20 to 30 seconds per yolk and about 30 seconds to 1 minute per white. Let stand, covered, about 2 minutes. Cool long enough to handle, then chop or chill until ready to use.

SAFETY OF EGG-CONTAINING DISHES

Salmonella will not survive in dishes cooked to 140°F (60°C) for at least 3½ minutes or in those cooked to 160°F (80°C). Cook poached, fried, soft-cooked, and scrambled eggs until whites are completely coagulated and yolks begin to thicken. Cook omelets, frittatas, and French toast until no visible liquid remains. When serving infants or individuals who are elderly, ill, or immune compromised, cook all egg dishes thoroughly or use a pasteurized egg product.

WHIPPING PROPERTIES

Beaten egg whites provide the volume and texture of many baked products, puffy omelets, soufflés, and chiffon cakes. The volume of beaten egg whites can increase 6 to 8 times.

Fat inhibits foam formation, therefore separate yolks and whites carefully to avoid the presence of any yolk in the white. Use metal or glass bowls for beating whites. Plastic bowls cannot be rendered completely fat free.

Separate eggs when cold, just out of the refrigerator. Let egg whites reach room temperature before whipping. Egg white foams should be beaten just until whites no longer slip when the bowl is tilted. Under-beaten whites result in poor volume of the finished product. Over-beaten whites have lost their elasticity and break apart when combined with other ingredients.

Drainage occurs fairly rapidly so whites should not be beaten more than a few minutes before they are needed.

Adding ⅛ teaspoon (0.5 ml) cream of tartar per egg white helps to stabilize the foam.

Sugar should be beaten in 1 or 2 teaspoons (5 or 10 ml) at a time after foaming has begun.

Beaten whole egg or egg yolk will increase about four times in volume. Beat until eggs become lemon-colored and form ribbons when beater is lifted, about three to five minutes. Egg yolks cannot be overbeaten as whites can be.

EGG PRODUCTS

In 1995, the Food Safety and Inspection Service (FSIS) became responsible for inspection of egg products. Processed and convenience forms of eggs available to food service include refrigerated liquid, frozen, dried (egg solids), and specialty products. All egg products are produced in federally inspected plants and are pasteurized so they are free of *Salmonella*.

Retail markets carry egg substitutes, in which yolks are replaced with oil, dried milk, gums, or other ingredients. Dried whole eggs usually are available at camping goods stores, and meringue powder, based on dried egg white, is available at craft stores because it is frequently used to frost baked goods. All such egg products are pasteurized (1970 Egg Products Inspection Act). Equivalency of large shell eggs to frozen, refrigerated liquid, and dried egg products is shown in Table 6.8 and Table 6.9.

TABLE 6.8

LARGE SHELL EGG EQUIVALENCY TO FROZEN OR REFRIGERATED LIQUID EGG PRODUCTS

		Weight		Measure	
Whole eggs	1	1¾ oz	50 g	3 Tbsp	45 ml
	10	1 lb 1¾ oz	503 g	2 cups	473 ml
	12	1 lb 5½ oz	610 g	2½ cups	592 ml
	25	2 lbs 13 oz	1276 g	1 qt 1¼ cups	1242 ml
	50	5 lbs 8 oz	2495 g	2 qt 2½ cups	2483 ml
Yolks	10	7¼ oz	206 g	¾ cup	177 ml
	12	8½ oz	241 g	¾ cup 2 Tbsp	207 ml
	22	1 lb	454 g	2 cups less 2 Tbsp	443 ml
Whites	10	11½ oz	326 g	1¼ cups 2 Tbsp	326 ml
	12	14 oz	397 g	1½ cups 2 Tbsp	385 ml
	14	1 lb	454 g	2 cups less 1 Tbsp	458 ml

TABLE 6.9

SHELL EGG EQUIVALENCY TO DRIED WHOLE EGG PRODUCTS

Shell Egg (Large Size)		Dried Whole Sifted		Water	
6	3 oz	85 g	1 cup	237 ml	1 cup
12	6 oz	170 g	2 cups	473 ml	2 cups
24	12 oz	340 g	1 qt	946 ml	1 qt
50	1 lb	709 g	2 qt	1971 ml	2 qt ⅓ cup
100	3 lb	1418 g	1 gal ⅔ cup	3942 ml	1 gal ⅔ cup
150	4 lb	2126 g	6 qt 1 cup	5915 ml	6 qt 1 cup
200	6 lb	2835 g	2 gal 1⅓ cup	7886 ml	2 gal 1⅓ cup

HANDLING EGG PRODUCTS

Do not accept frozen egg products that are beginning to thaw. Transfer frozen products to the freezer immediately after delivery.

Do not thaw at room temperature. Thaw in the refrigerator or under cold running water in sealed containers. Use defrosted egg products promptly. Cover and refrigerate unused portion and use within three days.

Refrigerate liquid egg products immediately upon delivery. Liquid product will keep, refrigerated at 40°F (4°C) or below and unopened, up to six days. Once opened, use immediately.

Store dried egg products in a dark cool (below 70°F, 20°C) place, preferably in the refrigerator.

Reconstitute only the amount of dried eggs that will be used immediately. Sift before measuring.

After opening dried eggs, seal tightly for re-storage and keep below 50°F (10°C).

Keep specialty egg products refrigerated or frozen according to their requirements.

TABLE 6.10
EGG STORAGE CHART

Product	Refrigerator	Freezer
Raw eggs in shell	3 to 5 weeks	Do not freeze. Instead, beat yolks and whites together; then freeze
Raw egg whites	2 to 4 days	12 months
Raw egg yolks	2 to 4 days	Yolks do not freeze well
Raw egg accidentally frozen in shell	Use immediately after thawing	Keep frozen; then refrigerate to thaw
Hard-cooked eggs	1 week	Do not freeze
Egg substitutes, liquid unopened	10 days	12 months
Egg substitutes, liquid opened	3 days	Do not freeze
Egg substitutes, frozen unopened	After thawing, 7 days or refer to "Use-By" date	12 months
Egg substitutes, frozen opened	After thawing, 3 days or refer to "Use-By" date	Do not freeze
Casseroles with eggs	3 to 4 days	After baking, 2 to 3 months
Eggnog, commercial	3 to 5 days	6 months
Eggnog, homemade	2 to 4 days	Do not freeze
Pies, pumpkin or pecan	3 to 4 days	After baking, 1 to 2 months
Pies, custard and chiffon	3 to 4 days	Do not freeze
Quiche with filling	3 to 4 days	After baking, 1 to 2 months

CHAPTER 7: Fruits

Fruits are produced from flowers and are the ripened ovaries and adjacent tissue of plants. Botanically, tomatoes, beans, eggplant, peppers, and some nuts are fruits, but in ordinary thinking, they are not.

The primary energy nutrient in fruits is carbohydrate, which occurs mainly as sugars. Fruits are also a valuable component in the diet due to their vitamin, mineral, phytochemical, and fiber content. Many fruits also contain high amounts of vitamins A and C.

Fruit consumption is increasing in the United States but is still below the recommended levels. Many varieties of fresh fruits are available year-round in almost every part of the United States because of excellent transportation and storage facilities, as well as increasing imports of exotic fruits.

FRESH FRUITS

CLASSIFICATION OR KINDS OF FRUITS

Fruits may be classified in a variety of different ways—by their appearance or substance, by the manner in which they are formed, by the chemical composition, or by ordinary usage.

One of the simplest classifications of fruits is the distinction between fleshy and dry fruits. Fleshy fruits are made of living cells and are often juicy and sweet. Dry fruits at maturity are made up of dead cells and are divided into those that split open and those that do not. Some nuts are included in this classification.

Fruits may be classified by the manner in which they are formed: simple fruits, aggregate fruits, or multiple fruits. A simple fruit is derived from a single pistil, or ovary, of a plant such as a plum or peach. Aggregate fruits are formed by the fusion of several separate pistils of one flower such as the blackberry, raspberry, or strawberry. Multiple fruits are formed by the fusion of several separate pistils of several grouped flowers. Multiple fruits include the pineapple, mulberry, and breadfruit.

A third manner of classification is based on chemical composition. Alkaline fruits include some apples, persimmons, sweet grapes, figs, dates, raisins, prunes, apricots, peaches, bananas, cherries, lychees, carob, and all dried fruits. Subacidic fruits include sweet apples, such as delicious, sweet peaches, sweet nectarines, pears, sweet cherries, papayas, mangoes, sweet plums, blueberries, raspberries, blackberries, mulberries, and huckleberries. Acid fruits are oranges, grapefruit, pineapples, strawberries, pomegranates, lemons, kiwi, kumquats, loquats, loganberries, gooseberries, cranberries, limes, sour apples, sour grapes, sour peaches, sour nectarines, sour plums, and sour cherries. Melons are classified as a separate group.

Most commonly, however, fruits are divided according to use rather than by any botanical classifications. Fruits may be classified as follows:

Berries — Those commonly marketed are blackberries, blueberries, boysenberries, cranberries, currants, elderberries, gooseberries, raspberries, and strawberries. Grapes, such as red flame and Thompson, seedless grapes, are a subcategory of berries.

Citrus — These are the grapefruits, kumquats, lemons, limes, mandarins, oranges, tangerines, and tangelos.

Drupes or stonefruits — This is the botanical name given to apricots, cherries, nectarines, peaches, and plums.

Melons — These vine-grown fruits include cantaloupe, casaba, Crenshaw, honeydew, and watermelon.

Pomes — These fruits include apples, pears, prickly pears, and quinces.

Tropical and semi-tropical — There are many species of tropical and semi-tropical fruits but those that are marketed commonly throughout the United States are avocados, bananas, coconuts, dates, figs, guavas, kiwis, mangoes, papayas, passion fruit, and pineapples.

Exotic — The more exotic fruits include persimmons, pomegranates, figs, guavas, Asian pear, atemoya, breadfruit, canistel, carambola (star fruit), cherimoya (custard apple), feijoa, gooseberries, longans, lychees, mangosteens, monstera, passion fruit (granadilla), quince, tamarinds, and ugli fruit.

PURCHASING

Fresh fruits have not been subjected to processing. They may be ripe or unripe, depending on their condition when harvested or the condition under which they have been stored. To utilize fresh fruits to the fullest benefit, careful purchasing choices must be made. The size of the fruit, its grade or quality, ripeness on delivery, and nutritional content may affect the use of the fruit.

Fresh fruits are sold by weight or count and are packed in various containers such as crates, bushels, cartons, cases, lugs, or flats.

Some fresh fruits are available trimmed, cleaned, peeled, or cut. Sugar and preservatives are sometimes added to these prepackaged, prepared fruits. The purchase price is often higher than it is for unpackaged fruits and the flavor, freshness, and nutritional qualities may suffer from the processing.

Sizes

Fruits sold in quantity are usually sold by weight or count rather than size. Medium sizes tend to be more desirable than very large, which often lack quality, or very small, which have little edible portion compared to wasted parts. At retail, many fruits that used to be sold by number may now be sold by weight. With the development in biotechnology, some fruits have been downsized to create miniatures, such as melons.

Grades

Grades of fresh fruits are established by the USDA's Agricultural Marketing Service (AMS) and used primarily in wholesale channels of distribution. They have been widely used by growers, shippers, and car lot receivers for domestic and foreign shipment but have not been used as extensively in the retail trade as those for canned products, which are packed in consumer-size containers. However, consumers have made considerable use of U.S. grades in the purchase of commodities such as apples, grapefruit, oranges, and peaches. These voluntary grades frequently are found on boxes of fresh fruit.

Most fruits purchased for food service operations and for retail sale are graded as U.S. Fancy. Fruits with lower grades are suitable for processing into sauces, jams, jellies, or preserves. Tropical fruits currently are not marketed under U.S. grades.

RIPENING FRUITS

Important changes take place in fruit as it ripens. The fruit reaches its full size, the pulp or flesh becomes soft and tender, and its color changes. Additionally, the acid level decreases, making it less tart, and its starch converts into the sugars fructose and glucose, providing a sweeter taste and aroma.

Depending upon the fruit, fresh fruits may be purchased either fully ripened or unripened. Some fruits such as figs and pineapples ripen only on the plant. Therefore, they must be harvested at or just before peak ripeness and rushed to the marketplace because they will never achieve full flavor or texture after they have been picked. Other fruits like bananas and pears continue to ripen after they have been harvested and may be purchased in an unripened state.

Ripening time and maintenance of fruit at its peak of freshness can be manipulated. Ripening can be delayed by chilling the fruit, which slows down the respiration rate. Slower respiration results in the slower conversion of starch to sugar. For quicker ripening, fruit can be stored at room temperature. Ripening also is affected by ethylene gas. Ethylene gas is emitted by ripening fruits and can be used to ripen most fruits further. Apples, tomatoes, melons, and bananas give off the most ethylene and should be stored away from other, more delicate fruits and vegetables. Fruits that have been picked unripened may be exposed to ethylene gas just prior to sale to speed up the ripening process. To extend the life of ripe fruits for a day or two, isolate them from other fruits or chill them. Special bags that release ethylene gas are now being marketed to extend the life of fresh fruits and vegetables.

Fresh fruits will not ripen further once they have been cooked or processed, however the cooking or processing method may soften or add flavor to the fruits.

PREPARING FRUITS

Most fruits are edible in a raw state and typically are served that way. When preparing fresh fruits for consumption, they should be washed thoroughly and peeled, sliced, or trimmed as needed. Some fruits can be washed well before use and stored, but some should not be washed until they are ready to be eaten. Fruits such as apples and bananas will brown once they are cut and should be dipped in lemon juice, pineapple juice, or a solution of vitamin C (including lemon-lime soda).

Some fruits can be cooked before eating. Commonly used cooking methods include broiling or grilling, baking, sauteing, deep-frying, poaching, simmering, and preserving. Proper care and attention must be given when cooking fruits because even minimal cooking can cause fruits to become extremely and irreversibly soft and mushy. To maintain the shape of a fruit, sugar or sugar syrup can be added. The sugar is absorbed slowly into the cell structure of the fruit, thus firming the fruit. Acids, like lemon juice, also can help cooked fruits retain their structure. If a fruit sauce is desired, cook the fruit in water to facilitate the disintegration of the tissues.

Dry-heat cooking methods include broiling or grilling, baking, sauteing, and deep-frying. Fruits are broiled or grilled just long enough to caramelize the sugar in them. They must be cooked quickly to preserve the structure of the fruit. Good fruits to broil and grill are pineapples, apples, grapefruits, banana, tomatoes, persimmons, and peaches. Fruits with sturdy skins like apples and pears can be baked after washing, coring or pitting, and peeling (if desired). Other fruit desserts are simple fruits that have been topped with a crust, crumbs, or batter and then baked. Fruits develop a rich, syrupy flavor when sauteed for short amounts of time in butter, sugar, and spices. Cherries, bananas, apples, pears, and pineapple are good choices for this method. Not all fruits are suitable for deep-frying. Apples, bananas, pears, pineapples, and firm peaches may be coated or mixed in a batter (fritters) and fried to produce pleasing results. Fruits may need to be dried thoroughly with paper towels so that the batter or coating will adhere to the fruit.

Moist-heat cooking methods include poaching and simmering. Poaching is one of the more popular cooking methods for fruits. Fruits are cooked slowly in low temperature liquids that allow them to soften gradually. Simmering techniques are used to make stewed fruits and compotes.

STORAGE AND USE

One of the greatest challenges that cooks face is keeping the kitchen stocked with fresh produce. Many fruits and vegetables begin to lose quality quickly once they have been harvested. Flavor, color, aroma, nutritional value, and texture all decline as produce ages. Fruits should be in good condition at the time of purchase, free of bruises, mold, brown or soft spots, and pest damage. They should have colors and textures that are appropriate to their type. They should be plump and not shriveled; any attached leaves should not be wilted.

The following storage guidelines will help to prolong the life and quality of fresh fruits:

- Most fresh produce should be stored under refrigeration with a few exceptions such as bananas and tomatoes.

- Fruits that need further ripening like peaches and avocados should be stored at room temperature until desired ripeness is reached and then refrigerated to slow down the ripening process.

- Storage temperatures for fresh fruits should be kept between 40–45°F with humidity levels of 80–90 percent.

- Keep fruits dry; excess moisture promotes spoilage.

- Store fruits that emit high amounts of ethylene gas, such as apples and melons, away from other produce because they will accelerate the ripening of those products. Lemons and melons also give off odors that can permeate other foods and should be stored separately.

- Refrigerate ripe stonefruits/drupes uncovered and plan to use within three to five days.

- Coat cut fruit with lemon juice or ascorbic acid to avoid discoloration of pared apples, peaches, bananas, and avocados, which occurs when the pared fruits are exposed to air.

- Most tropical fruits will soften at room temperature, giving slightly to pressure when ripe. Ripe fruit needs to be refrigerated.

PROCESSED FRUITS

Many fruits are available in frozen, canned, dried, and dehydrated forms. The number and kinds of processed foods available at the retail market are constantly increasing as new procedures and equipment are developed for processing foods of improved quality. Their convenience and availability year-round have added variety to menus, particularly in the winter.

FROZEN AND CANNED FRUITS

Canned fruit is cooked fruit that has been sealed and processed for keeping. Some fruits such as cherries and berries are commonly frozen. Frozen fruits to be used raw should be barely defrosted when served so the fruit will not become excessively soft prior to use. Standards of identity for most canned fruits as well as minimum standards of quality for many of the principal ones have been established by the U.S. Food and Drug Administration. The U.S. Department of Agriculture has developed grade standards that also reflect factors of quality for any frozen and canned fruits. Canners, freezers, and distributors often voluntarily use the grade designation on their labels. Grades reflect mainly differences in appearance. The factors most important in evaluating the quality of processed fruits are flavor, color, texture, uniformity of size and shape, ripeness, and absence of defects. The permissive grades established by industry for most processed fruits are A (fancy), B (choice) or C (standard). The terms in parentheses are those in common commercial usage for designating the quality of processed products.

DRIED FRUITS

Apples, apricots, blueberries, cherries, figs, peaches, prunes, and raisins may be sun dried, mechanically dehydrated, vacuum dried, foam-mat dried, or explosively puffed. The moisture content of the dried fruits generally ranges from 15 to 25 percent. Quality levels or grades for most dried fruit are the same as they are for other fruits. The sizes of dried fruit—small, medium, large, extra-large, or jumbo—appear on retail packages. Dried fruits may be soaked in water to rehydrate prior to cooking. The higher sugar content of dried fruits makes the use of more sugar for sweetening undesirable.

TABLE 7.1
FRESH FRUIT BUYING GUIDE

Varieties	What To Look For	What To Avoid	Additional Information
Apples			
Apple variations for eating out of hand or in salads or fruit cups include Delicious, Gala, Golden Delicious, Jonathan, Macintosh, Spartans, Stayman, and Winesap. The tart and slightly acid apples—Granny Smith, Gravenstein, Grimes Golden, Jonathan, and Newton—are excellent for pies and sauces. Firm-fleshed apples that hold shape well in baking include Northern Spy, Rhode Island Greening, Rome Beauty, Winesap, and York Imperial.	Firm, well-colored fruit. Apples must be mature when picked to have good flavor, crisp texture and storing ability.	Immature apples that lack color for the particular variety; fruit with shriveled skin; overripe apples (indicated by a yielding to slight pressure on the skin and soft mealy flesh); and apples affected by freezing (indicated by internal breakdown and bruised areas). Scald on apples (irregularly shaped tan or brown areas) may not seriously affect the eating quality of the apple.	Store late-maturing apple varieties, like Jonathan and Red Delicious, for 3 to 5 months if they are harvested at peak ripeness without bruising. Refrigerate immediately after picking at 30 to 32°F with 90% humidity. Perforated plastic bags will allow for some air circulation. Coat cut fruit with lemon juice or ascorbic acid to avoid discoloration of pared apples.
Apricots			
Many varieties with different harvest times from mid-spring to late summer/early fall.	Apricots that are plump and juicy looking and have a uniform, golden-orange color. Ripe apricots will yield to gentle pressure on the skin.	Dull-looking, soft or mushy fruit, and very firm, pale yellow or greenish yellow fruit. These are indications of over-maturity or immaturity, respectively.	Fresh apricots come to market from mid-spring to mid-summer, May through July, and even later in the Northern Hemisphere. The apricot harvest can be divided into early, mid-season, and late. That means one can enjoy some or all of these over the course of the apricot harvest.

FRESH FRUIT BUYING GUIDE (CONTINUED)

Varieties	What To Look For	What To Avoid	Additional Information
Avocados			
Mexican Variety Avocados (includes Zutano, Bacon, Fuerte). The Mexican avocado varieties tend to be pear shaped, smooth in skin, and green in color. On average they have a lower fat content. Guatemalan Variety Avocados (includes Hass, Pinkerton, Reed, and Gwen). The Guatemalan varieties of avocado tend to have a thicker and sometimes pebbly skin with a rounder shape. Their fruit tends to be higher in fat.	For immediate use, slightly soft avocados that yield to a gentle pressure on the skin. For use in a few days, firm fruits that do not yield to the squeeze test. Irregular light brown markings are sometimes found on the outside skin. These markings have no effect on the flesh of the avocado.	Avocados with dark sunken spots in irregular patches or cracked or broken surfaces. These are signs of decay.	Leave them at room temperature to ripen and refrigerate once desired ripeness is reached.
Bananas			
Bananas generally fall under the categories of either sweet dessert bananas or starchy and best for cooking. More than 1,000 banana varieties exist throughout the world. The most well-known variety of sweet dessert bananas is the Cavendish banana. Many people call the starchy type of bananas "plantains" instead of bananas.	Bananas that are firm, bright in appearance, and free from bruises or other injury. The stage of ripeness is indicated by the skin color; best eating quality has been reached when the solid yellow color is specked with brown. At this stage, the flesh is mellow and the flavor is fully developed. Bananas with green tips or with practically no yellow color have not developed their full flavor potential.	Bruised fruit (which means rapid deterioration and waste); discolored skins (a sign of decay); a dull, grayish, aged appearance (showing that the bananas have been exposed to cold and will not ripen properly). Occasionally, the skin may be entirely brown and yet the flesh will still be in prime condition. Flavor will be fully developed.	Keep bananas at room temperature until ripe and then refrigerate. Bananas do not ripen normally if chilled before fully ripe. Cold temperatures darken the skins, but will not affect palatability. Bananas are first in fruit sales in the United States.

FRESH FRUIT BUYING GUIDE (CONTINUED)

Varieties	What To Look For	What To Avoid	Additional Information
Berries			
Berries should be washed just before use. Berries will mold and spoil more rapidly if washed before storage.			
Blueberries	A dark blue color with a silvery bloom, which is a natural, protective waxy coating; blueberries that are plump, firm, uniform, dry, and free from stems or leaves.	Soft, mushy berries; berries with broken skins; moldy berries.	Maine produces 25% of all low-bush blueberries in North America, making it the largest producer in the world
Cranberries	Plump, firm berries with a lustrous color for the best quality. Duller varieties should at least have some red color.	Occasional soft, spongy, or leaky berries should be sorted out before cooking because they may produce an off-flavor.	About 95% of cranberries are processed into products such as juice drinks, sauce, and sweetened dried cranberries. The remaining 5% are sold fresh to consumers.
Blackberries Boysenberries Gooseberries Loganberries Raspberries	A bright, clean appearance and a uniform good color for the species. The individual small cells making up the berry should be plump and tender but not mushy. Look for berries that are fully ripened and with no attached stem caps.	Leaky and moldy berries. Also note wet or stained spots on wood or fiber containers; these are possible signs of poor quality or spoiled berries.	Brambles are the name for those fruiting plants that have thorns, such as raspberries, blackberries, dewberries, boysenberries, and gooseberries. These fruits are hard to ship, so buy them locally or grow them if fresh berries are desired.
Strawberries	Berries with a full red color and a bright luster, firm flesh, and the cap stem still attached. The berries should be dry and clean; usually medium to small strawberries have better eating qualities than do the larger berries.	Berries with large uncolored areas or with large seedy areas (poor in flavor and texture), a dull shrunken appearance or softness (sign of decay), or those with mold, which can spread rapidly from one berry to another.	When purchasing strawberries, pick the most fragrant berries. Strawberries do not ripen after they have been harvested, so choose berries that have been picked fully ripe.

FRESH FRUIT BUYING GUIDE (CONTINUED)

Varieties	What To Look For	What To Avoid	Additional Information
Cherries			
Cherries may be of the sweet variety for eating out of hand or they may be tart, sometimes called sour cherries, and used in cooking and baking. These are lighter red in color than the sweet cherries and have a softer flesh. Most of the commercial crop of tart cherries goes to processors.	A very dark color is the most important indication of good flavor and maturity in sweet cherries. Bing, Tartarian, Chapman, Black, Republican, and Schmidt varieties should range from deep maroon to mahogany red to black, for richer flavor. Lambert cherries should be dark red. Good cherries have bright, glossy, plump-looking surfaces and fresh looking stems.	Over-mature cherries lacking in flavor, indicated by shriveling, dried stems, and a generally dull appearance. Decay is fairly common on sweet cherries, but because of the normal dark color, decayed areas often are inconspicuous. Soft, leaking fruit, brown discoloration, and mold growth are indications of decay.	Cherries have a very short growing season and can grow in most temperate latitudes. The peak season for cherries is in the summer.
Citrus Fruits			
Store citrus fruits—except tangerines—in the refrigerator uncovered.			
Grapefruits Grapefruit may be white- or pink-fleshed, with or without seeds.	Firm, well-shaped fruits—heavy for their size—are usually the best eating. Thin-skinned fruits have more juice than coarse-skinned ones. If a grapefruit is pointed at the stem end, it is likely to be thick-skinned. Rough, rigid, or wrinkled skin can also be an indication of thick skin and lack of juice. Grapefruit often has skin defects—such as scale, scars, thorn scratches, or discoloration—which usually do not affect the eating quality.	Soft, discolored areas on the peel at the stem end; water-soaked areas; loss of bright color; and soft and tender peel that breaks easily with finger pressure. These are all symptoms of decay, which has an objectionable effect on flavor.	Tangelo is a hybrid of a tangerine or mandarin orange and a grapefruit or pomelo.

FRESH FRUIT BUYING GUIDE (CONTINUED)

Varieties	What To Look For	What To Avoid	Additional Information
Citrus Fruits (continued)			
Lemons	Lemons with a rich yellow color, reasonably smooth-textured skin with a slight gloss, and those that are firm and heavy. A pale or greenish yellow color means very fresh fruit with slightly higher acidity. Coarse or rough skin texture is a sign of thick skin and not much flesh.	Lemons with a darker yellow or dull color, or with hardening or shriveling of the skin (sign of age) and those with soft spots, mold on the surface, and punctures of the skin (sign of decay).	Lemons can be kept for weeks in the home refrigerator if placed in a jar with a tight-fitting lid to prevent loss of moisture.
Limes Limes may be available in two basic varieties. The Persian, or Tahiti, lime is rounder, larger, and thinner skinned than the Key lime (Mexican or West Indies lime).	Limes with a glossy skin and heavy weight for the size.	Limes with full, dry skin (a sign of aging and loss of acid flavor), and those showing evidence of decay (soft spots, mold and skin puncture).	As limes ripen, they become yellow and less acidic.
Oranges Orange varieties include Navel from California and Arizona; Valencia from California, Arizona, Florida, and Texas; and mandarins. Mandarins include satsumas, tangerines, and miscellaneous hybrids, such as Temple oranges from Florida, a cross between a tangerine and an orange. Murcott is a cross between a sweet orange and a mandarin.	Firm and heavy oranges with fresh, bright-looking skin that is reasonably smooth for the variety.	Lightweight oranges, which are likely to lack flesh content and juice. Very rough skin texture indicates abnormally thick skin and less flesh. Dull, dry skin and spongy texture indicate aging and deteriorated eating quality. Also avoid decay—shown by cuts or skin punctures, soft spots on the surface, and discolored, weakened areas of skin around the stem end or button.	Tangelo is a hybrid of a tangerine or mandarin orange and a grapefruit or pomelo.

FRESH FRUIT BUYING GUIDE (CONTINUED)

Varieties	What To Look For	What To Avoid	Additional Information
Citrus Fruits (continued)			
Tangerines	Deep yellow or orange color and a bright luster are the best signs of fresh, mature, good-flavored tangerines. Because of the typically loose nature of the tangerine skin, they will frequently not feel firm to the touch.	Very pale yellow or greenish fruits, likely to be lacking in flavor (although small green areas on otherwise high-colored fruits are not bad) and tangerines with cut or punctured skins or very soft spots (all signs of decay, which spreads rapidly).	Tangelo is a hybrid of a tangerine or mandarin orange and a grapefruit or pomelo. Place tangerines in a plastic bag for refrigerator storage.
Grapes			
The European varieties of grapes include Cardinal (early bright red), Emperor (late deep red), Ribier (late black), Thompson seedless (early green), and Tokay (late red). The American varieties include Catawba, Concord (blue-black), Delaware, and Niagara. Varietal groups include table, raisin, wine, juice, and canning.	Well-colored plump grapes that are firmly attached to the stem. White or green grapes are sweetest when the color has a yellowish cast or straw color, with a tinge of amber. Red varieties are better when a good red predominates on all or most of the berries. Bunches are more likely to hold together if the stems are green and pliable. Grapes will not improve in sweetness, quality, or color after picking.	Soft or wrinkled grapes (showing effects of freezing or drying), grapes with bleached areas around the stem end (indicating injury and poor quality), and grapes leaking brownish fluid (a sign of decay).	Approximately 71% of world grape production is used for wine, 27% as fresh fruit, and 2% as dried fruit.
Kiwi/Kiwifruit			
Chinese New Zealand California	Kiwifruit is ripe when it yields to gentle pressure. To ripen, place hard fruit in a plastic bag with an apple or banana for 1 to 2 days at room temperature.	Soft, dark areas, indentations, broken skin, uneven color.	Firm kiwifruit ripen after a few days to a week when stored at room temperature, but should not be kept in direct sunlight. Faster ripening occurs when placed in a paper bag with an apple, pear, or banana.

FRESH FRUIT BUYING GUIDE (CONTINUED)

Varieties	What To Look For	What To Avoid	Additional Information
Melons			

Melons are among the most difficult fruits to select. A characteristic aroma and color with heaviness in relation to size are indicators of good quality. Good food handling practices, including washing of melons before cutting, should be followed when preparing melons.

Varieties	What To Look For	What To Avoid	Additional Information
Cantaloupe (Muskmelon) / Persian Melon	Three major signs of full maturity: 1. The stem should be gone, leaving a smooth, symmetrical, shallow basin called a "full-slip." If all or part of the stem base remains or if the stem scar is jagged or torn, the melon is probably not fully matured. 2. The netting, or veining, should be thick, coarse, and corky and should stand out in bold relief over some part of the surface. 3. The skin color (ground color) between the netting should have changed from green to a yellowish buff, yellowish gray, or pale yellow. Look for signs of ripeness—a cantaloupe may be mature, but not ripe. A ripe cantaloupe will have a yellowish cast to the rind, have a pleasant cantaloupe odor when held to the nose, and will yield slightly to light thumb pressure on the blossom end of the melon.	Over-ripeness, shown by a pronounced yellow rind color, a softening over the entire rind, and soft, watery, and insipid flesh. Small bruises normally will not hurt the fruit, but large bruised areas should be avoided because they generally cause soft, water-soaked areas underneath the rind. Mold growth on the cantaloupe—particularly in the stem scar with wet tissue under the mold—indicates decay.	To ripen cantaloupe, let stand at room temperature 2 to 4 days. Chill a few hours in refrigerator before serving. Melons stored in the refrigerator should be used within a week. Persian melon resembles cantaloupe but is nearly round, has finer netting, and is similar in size to honeydew.

FRESH FRUIT BUYING GUIDE (CONTINUED)

Varieties	What To Look For	What To Avoid	Additional Information
Melons (continued)			
Casaba	Ripe melons with a gold yellow rind color and a slight softening at the blossom end. Casabas have no odor or aroma.	Decayed melons, shown by dark, sunken water-soaked spots.	Casaba melon is pumpkin shaped and has no netting but does have shallow, irregular, lengthwise furrows.
Crenshaw	A deep golden yellow rind, sometimes with small areas of a lighter shade of yellow; a surface that yields slightly to moderate pressure of the thumb, particularly at the blossom end; a pleasant aroma.	Slightly sunken, water-soaked areas on the rind (a sign of decay, which spreads quickly through the melon).	A Crenshaw melon is a hybrid melon with very sweet, juicy orange flesh. Crenshaws are among the sweetest of melons.
Honeyball / Honeydew	Maturity, shown by a soft, velvety feel, and for ripeness, shown by a slight softening at the blossom end, a faint pleasant fruit aroma, and a yellowish white to cream rind color.	Melons with a dead-white or greenish white color and hard, smooth feel, bruised areas (sign of injury), and cuts or punctures through the rind (leads to decay). Small, superficial, sunken spots do not damage the melon for immediate use but large decayed spots will.	Honeydew melon is large, bluntly oval, and smooth. Santa Claus, or Christmas, melons look like small watermelons with the flesh of a honeydew.
Watermelon	In cut melons, firm, juicy flesh with good red color, free of white streaks; seeds that are dark brown or black. In whole melons, a relatively smooth surface, neither shiny nor dull, ends that are rounded and filled out; creamy colored underside.	Melons with pale-colored flesh, and white streaks or "white heart," (whitish seeds indicating immaturity). Dry, mealy flesh or watery, stringy flesh are signs of over-maturity or aging after harvest.	Santa Claus, or Christmas, melons look like small watermelons with the flesh of a honeydew.

FRESH FRUIT BUYING GUIDE (CONTINUED)

Varieties	What To Look For	What To Avoid	Additional Information
Nectarines			
Like peaches, nectarine varieties may be either freestone or clingstone.	Rich color and plumpness and a slight softening along the "seam" of the nectarine. Most varieties have an orange-yellow color (ground color) between the red areas, but some varieties have a greenish ground color. Bright-looking fruits that are firm to moderately hard will probably ripen normally within 2 to 3 days at room temperature.	Hard, dull fruits or slightly shriveled fruits (which may be immature—picked too soon—and of poor eating quality), and soft to overripe fruits or those with cracked or punctured skin or other signs of decay. Russeting or staining of the skin may affect the appearance but not detract from the internal quality of the nectarine.	The nectarine got its start in China as a genetic variant of the common peach and is not, as some believe, the consequence of a cross between a peach and a plum. One Chinese emperor was so enthralled with nectarines that he and his people referred to them as the "nectar of the gods."
Peaches			
Peach varieties are divided into freestone (Elberta, O'Henry, and Redtop) and clingstone (Flavorcrest, June Lady, Red Haven, and Springcrest). As the names imply, the flesh of the freestone peach separates readily from the pit, whereas the reverse is true of the clingstone. In general, freestones are preferred for eating fresh and for freezing. Both kinds may be canned, but the clingstone maintains the firmer shape.	Peaches that are fairly firm or are becoming a trifle soft. The skin color between the red areas (ground color) should be yellow or at least creamy with a peachy fragrance.	Very firm or hard peaches with a distinctly green ground color, which are probably immature and will not ripen properly. Also avoid very soft fruits, which are overripe. Do not buy peaches with large flattened bruises (they will have areas of discolored flesh underneath) or peaches with any sign of decay. Decay starts as a pale tan spot that expands in a circle and gradually turns darker in color.	

FRESH FRUIT BUYING GUIDE (CONTINUED)

Varieties	What To Look For	What To Avoid	Additional Information
Pears			
Bartlett pears, Forelle, and Seckel are summer and early fall pears that are eaten fresh and are used in canning. Fall and winter pear varieties include Bosc, D'Anjou, Comice, and Winter Nellis. These keep well in cold storage.	Firm pears of all varieties. The color depends on variety. For Bartletts, look for a pale yellow to rich yellow color; Bosc—greenish yellow to brownish yellow (the brown cast is caused by skin russeting, a characteristic of the Bosc pear); D'Anjou or Comice— light green to yellowish green; Winter Nellis—medium to light green. Pears that are hard when purchased will probably ripen if kept at room temperature, but it is wise to select pears that have already begun to soften to be reasonably sure that they will ripen satisfactorily.	Wilted or shriveled pears with dull-appearing skin and slight weakening of the flesh near the stem, which indicates immaturity. These pears will not ripen. Also avoid spots on the sides or blossom ends of the pear, which means that corky tissue may be underneath.	Pick pears when still slightly green and firm. Refrigerate at 30–35°F for 1 to 3 months. To ripen, place at room temperature for 1 week. To ripen faster, seal pears in plastic bag; accumulated ethylene gas will hasten the process. The most popular type of pear is the Bartlett. Pears are generally firm when purchased, but will soften at room temperature.
Plums/prunes			
Plums may be red, green, or purplish yellow. Prunes are a variety of freestone plums suitable for drying; they are purplish-black, smaller, and more oval than other types of plums.	Plums and prunes with a good color for the variety, in a fairly firm to slightly soft stage of ripeness.	Fruits with skin breaks, punctures, or brownish discoloration. Also avoid immature fruits (relatively hard, poorly colored, very tart, sometimes shriveled) and over-mature fruits (excessively soft, possibly leaking or decaying).	The peak season for domestic plums is June through September. Plums should be slightly soft when ripe.

FRESH FRUIT BUYING GUIDE (CONTINUED)

Varieties	What To Look For	What To Avoid	Additional Information
Pineapples			
Red Spanish, Smooth Cayenne, Queen, and Natal pineapples are most common to American markets.	The color, the fragrant pineapple odor, a very slight separation of the eyes or pips, and the ease with which the "spikes" or leaves can be pulled out from the top. Pineapples are usually dark green in mature, hard stage. As the more popular varieties (such as Red Spanish and Smooth Cayenne) ripen, the green color fades and orange and yellow take its place. When fully ripe, the pineapples are golden yellow, orange yellow, or reddish brown—depending on the variety, although one seldom seen pineapple (the Sugar Loaf) remains green even when ripe. Also look for maturity, shown by plump glossy eyes or pips, firmness, a lively color, and fruits that are heavy for their size. A ripe pineapple will spring back slightly when touched.	Pineapples with sunken or slightly pointed pips, dull yellowish-green color, and dried appearance (all signs of immaturity). Also avoid bruised fruit (shown by discolored or soft spots), which are susceptible to decay. Other signs of decay (which spreads rapidly through the fruit) are traces of mild, unpleasant odor and eyes that turn watery and darken in color.	Pineapples are picked at the peak of ripeness and flavor; they do not ripen after harvest.

CHAPTER 8: Vegetables

FRESH VEGETABLES

Fresh vegetables are available throughout the year due to mass transportation and quality controlled storage. U.S. markets provide fresh vegetables from around the world. In our health-conscious times, vegetables are used not just as side dishes but also as an economical foundation for many main dishes. Vegetables are often used as the main food item for people embracing a vegetarian or vegan lifestyle. In addition to their nutritional value, vegetables contribute flavor, color, and texture to foods presented on the plate.

Daily intake should include three to five servings of vegetables (½ cup cooked or 1 cup of raw). Vegetables supply vitamins and minerals including Vitamins A and C, riboflavin, folic acid, iron, and magnesium. Most vegetables are high in fiber and low in cholesterol and fat.

CLASSIFICATION OR KINDS OF VEGETABLES

Vegetables are classified according to the portion of the plant that is eaten. The following classification is a general list; many more types and varieties are available worldwide.

Bulbs — Producing a fleshy, leafy shoot above the ground, bulbs usually consist of layers or clustered segments. Examples: onions, garlic, leeks, and shallots.

Flowers and fruits — Vegetable flowers are edible on certain plants and vegetable fruits are mature ovaries that contain seeds. Examples: artichoke, broccoli, cauliflower, cucumber, eggplant, fennel, okra, pepper, pumpkin, squash, corn, tomato, and water chestnuts.

Leaves and stems — The edible leaves and stalks of the plant when the stalk is the main part of the vegetable. Examples: asparagus, Brussels sprouts, cabbage, celery, Chinese cabbage, chives, greens, kale, kohlrabi, lettuce, parsley, seaweed, spinach, and watercress.

Legumes — The mature, dry seeds of the family *Fabaceae* or *Leguminosae* are usually obtained from pods. Sometimes the pods are eaten along with the seeds. Examples: adzuki, common beans, broadbean (*Vicia faba*), carob, chickpeas, cowpeas, hyacinth beans (dhal), lentils, lima beans, mung beans, mungo beans, peas, peanuts, soybeans, and winged beans.

Roots — These are usually a long or round-shaped taproot—literally the root of the plant itself. Examples: beet, carrot, cassava (manioc or tapioca), celeriac, daikon, jicama, kohlrabi, parsnip, radish, rutabaga, sweet potato, and turnip.

Tubers — These grow underground on the root of the plant, not the root itself. Examples: Jerusalem artichoke and Irish potato.

Fungi — When referring to vegetables, fungi are most commonly known as mushrooms and truffles.

Crucifers — Vegetables of the family *Brassicaceae* (also called *Cruciferae*) are called cruciferous vegetables. Vegetables of many different classifications come from this family. Crucifers may provide even more health benefits than other vegetables. Crucifers include bok choy, broccoli, Brussels sprouts, cabbage, cauliflower, collards, kale, kohlrabi, mustard greens, rutabagas, turnips, and their greens.

Notes:

The taro "bulb" used to make poi is the corm of the plant (not a bulb, not a root, and not a tuber). Corms are vertically thickened underground stems that store starch.

Bamboo shoots are also considered vegetables.

PURCHASING VEGETABLES

High quality, fresh vegetables are young, crisp, and brightly colored. The quality of fresh produce decreases with age, therefore it is best to buy them fresh and use within a week. Purchase fresh vegetables when in season for best quality and lowest prices. Look for local varieties because the shorter transportation allows for a fresher product. Local farmer's markets are an excellent choice for obtaining fresh, local produce. Handle fresh produce carefully. Bruised and damaged vegetables decay more rapidly.

Grades for Fresh Vegetables

U.S. grading standards for fresh vegetables are voluntary; the principal factors affecting the grade are maturity, decay, shipping quality, appearance, and waste caused by various defects. The U.S. No. 1 grade is designed to include a good proportion of the commercial crop. Standards for some commodities provide a "fancy grade" used by packers of superior vegetables for which a premium is obtained. U.S. No. 1 is the highest grade for most vegetables. Other fresh vegetable grades (No. 2 or Combination) are not likely to appear in retail stores.

PREPARING VEGETABLES

Because vegetables grow close to the ground, it is necessary to wash them carefully. It also may be necessary to scrape, pare, chop, or slice some vegetables before cooking. For most vegetables, maximum nutrition is obtained when eaten raw.

Cooking vegetables does lead to inevitable nutrient loss, so use cooking practices that will minimize the loss. Most minerals and some vitamins can be lost in water. Soaking vegetables in water before cooking or cooking them in large amounts of water causes leaching of important vitamins and minerals. Other factors that lead to nutrient loss are high temperatures, prolonged cooking, alkalis (such as baking soda and hard water), plant enzymes (which are destroyed by heat), and oxygen. Some nutrient loss is inevitable, but understanding how these factors affect vegetables can help to avoid much of the nutrient loss. Cooking also affects the texture, flavor, and color of vegetables.

Vegetables can be cooked by microwaving, steaming, baking/broiling, boiling, sauteing, frying, stir-frying, braising, or pressure-cooking. The length of time required for a given vegetable to cook by any method cannot be stated exactly. Cooking time differs with the variety and maturity of each vegetable, the period and the temperature at which the vegetable was held after it was harvested, and the size of the pieces. Each vegetable should be cooked for the shortest time necessary to give a palatable product.

BASIC COOKING METHODS

General Procedures

• Use as little water as possible, with the exception of strong-flavored vegetables.

• Cook vegetables as quickly as possible to soften fibers and retain nutrients, color, and flavor.

• Drain vegetables, but save the cooking water because it contains nutrients and flavor. Use the water in soups, sauces, and gravies.

• Season vegetables before serving. Use salt and high-fat sauces and butter sparingly.

Microwave Cookery

Vegetables cook quickly and easily in the microwave oven. Only a few tablespoons of water are needed and microwaving preserves the nutrients, color, and texture of most vegetables. Always cover vegetables in the microwave. To microwave vegetables:

Place evenly cut vegetables in a microwave-safe dish. Add 2 tablespoons of water to fresh vegetables. Frozen vegetables usually require no extra water.

Cover the vegetables and cook on high until fork tender. Halfway through the cooking cycle, stir the vegetables.

To microwave frozen vegetables, follow the package directions.

Allow approximately a 3-minute resting time after the recommended cooking time. Food continues to cook during this period.

STORAGE AND USE

• Store the following vegetables in refrigerator crisper or in a plastic bag in refrigerator: asparagus, beets, and broccoli. Brussels sprouts, beet greens, cabbage, carrots, cauliflower, celery, chard, collard greens, cucumber, green onions, lettuce, mushrooms, mustard greens, okra, peppers, spinach, summer squash, and turnip greens.

- Store sweet corn in husks, uncovered in refrigerator.

- Store ripe tomatoes, uncovered, in the refrigerator. Keep unripe tomatoes at room temperature, but away from direct sunlight until they ripen.

- Store dry onions in loosely woven or open mesh containers at room temperature or slightly cooler temperatures.

- Store potatoes in a dark, dry, well-ventilated place at temperatures between 45 and 50° F (7 and 10° C). Potatoes stored at room temperature need to be used sooner than those stored under ideal conditions to prevent greening or sprouting and shriveling.

- Store these vegetables at 60°F (15°C): hard rind squashes, eggplant, rutabagas, and sweet potatoes. Temperatures below 50° F (10° C) may cause chilling injury. If these vegetables must be kept at room temperature, plan to use them within a week.

- Use these vegetables within one or two days: asparagus, beet greens, broccoli, Brussels sprouts, chard, collard greens, green peas, green onions, kale, lettuce and other salad greens, fresh lima beans, mushrooms, mustard greens, spinach, sweet corn, and turnip greens.

PROCESSED VEGETABLES

CANNED AND FROZEN VEGETABLES

Vegetables may be frozen or canned separately or in combination with other vegetables. The different forms include whole, sliced, diced, mashed, puree, juice, and soup.

Grades for Canned and Frozen Vegetables

The Standards of Quality and Fill as outlined by FDA are minimal, basic requirements that serve as a pattern for good processing techniques for the commercial food processor. FDA Standards of Identity tell us what a product is.

The U.S. Grade Standards developed by USDA are essentially market classifications of quality. Processors are not required by law to include the grade on the label. The U.S. grade names are U.S. Grade A or Fancy, U.S. Grade B or Extra-Standard, and U.S. Grade C or Standard. The four quality characteristics used to determine the grade are color, uniformity of size, texture, and absence of defects. Additional grading factors that are used include consistency, clearness of liquid, size and symmetry, drained weight, wholeness, and flavor.

Storage of Canned and Frozen Vegetables

Store unopened canned vegetables in a cool, dry place. For best quality, use canned vegetables within a year of purchase. Vegetables lose quality and some nutrients if food is stored too long. Check all canned products to make sure the seal is not broken and the can is not bulging.

Frozen vegetables should be stored at 0°F (-18°C) or lower to retain quality and nutritive value for 8 to 12 months. Before buying large qualities of frozen vegetables, check the freezer or freezing compartment temperature. If the temperature is above 0°F (-18°C), plan to use frozen vegetables within a few days for best quality.

DRIED AND FREEZE-DRIED VEGETABLES

Dried and freeze-dried vegetables are readily available in markets. Health food and sporting goods sections in large stores typically carry a wide selection of dried and freeze-dried foods.

Storage of Dried Vegetables

Optimal storage conditions for dried foods are:

- Keep storage temperature below 60°F

- Store in clean, cool, dry, and dark storage area

- Use airtight and moisture-proof packaging

For best quality and nutritional value, dried foods should be used within one year of purchase.
Substituting Dried Foods for Fresh

Substitute reconstituted vegetable powders and flakes for finely chopped fresh vegetables in recipes. If you do not reconstitute the powders or flakes before adding them to the recipe ingredients, add a small amount of liquid to the recipe. Allow ¼ cup (60 ml) liquid for each tablespoon of powder and each 1½ tablespoons (23 ml) of flakes.

Substitute 1 tablespoon (15 ml) vegetable powder or ½ tablespoon vegetable flakes or 2 tablespoons (30 ml) dried pieces for 4 tablespoons (60 ml) chopped fresh vegetables.

TABLE 8.1
VEGETABLE BUYING GUIDE

Vegetable	What To Look For	What To Avoid
Artichokes	Plump, globular artichokes that are heavy in relation to size, and compact with thick, green, fresh-looking leaf scales. Size is not important in relation to quality.	Artichokes with large areas of brown on the scales and with spreading scales (a sign of age, indicating drying and toughening of the edible portions), grayish black discoloration (caused by bruises), mold growth on the scales, and worm injury
Asparagus	Closed, compact tips, smooth, round spears, and a fresh appearance. A rich green color should cover most of the spear. Stalks should be tender almost as far down as the green extends.	Tips that are open and spread out, moldy or decayed tips, ribbed spears (up and down ridges), or spears that are not rounded. These are signs of aging and indicate tough asparagus and poor flavor. Avoid excessively sandy asparagus because sand grains can lodge beneath the scales and are difficult to wash out.
Beans (snap beans)	A fresh, bright appearance with good color for the variety. Get young, tender beans with pods in firm crisp condition.	Wilted or flabby bean pods, serious blemishes, and decay. Thick, tough, fibrous pods indicate over-maturity.
Beets	Beets that are a rich, deep red color, firm, round, and smooth over most of the surface and have a slender tap root (the large main root). If beets are bunched, judge their freshness by the condition of the tops. Badly wilted or decayed tops indicate a lack of freshness, but the roots may be satisfactory if they are firm.	Elongated beets with round, scaly areas around the top surface; these will be tough, fibrous, and strong flavored. Avoid wilted, flabby beets that have been exposed to the air too long.
Broccoli	A firm, compact cluster of small flower buds, with none opened enough to show the bright yellow flower. Bud clusters should be dark green, sage green, or even green with a decidedly purplish cast. Stems should not be too thick or tough.	Broccoli with spread bud clusters, enlarged or open buds, yellowish green color, or wilted condition—signs of over-maturity and overlong display. Avoid broccoli with soft, slippery, water-soaked spots on the bud cluster. These are signs of decay.

VEGETABLE BUYING GUIDE (CONTINUED)

Vegetable	What To Look For	What To Avoid
Brussels Sprouts	A fresh, bright green color, tight fitting outer leaves, firm body, and free of blemishes.	Brussels sprouts with yellow or yellowish green leaves or leaves that are loose, soft, or wilted. Small holes or ragged leaves may indicate worm injury.
Cabbage	Cabbage may be red, green with smooth leaves, or green with crinkly leaves—a variety known as Savoy. Look for firm or hard heads of cabbage that are heavy for their size. Outer leaves should be a good green or red color (depending on type), reasonably fresh, and free from serious blemishes. The outer leaves (called "wrapper" leaves) fit loosely on the head and are usually discarded, but too many loose wrapper leaves on a head cause waste. With Savoy cabbage, look for crumpled leaves with developed round heads of dark green color. Some early crop cabbage may be soft or only fairly firm but is suitable for immediate use if the leaves are fresh and crisp. Cabbage that has been in storage is usually trimmed of all outer leaves and lacks color but is satisfactory if not wilted.	New cabbage with wilted or decayed outer leaves or with leaves turning yellow. Worm-eaten outer leaves often indicate that the worm injury penetrates into the head. Stored cabbage with outer leaves badly discolored, dried, or decayed probably is over-aged. Separation of the stems of leaves from the central stem at the base of the head also indicates over-age.
Carrots	Carrots that are well formed, smooth, well colored, and firm.	Roots with large, green sunburned areas at the top (which must be trimmed) and roots that are flabby from wilting or show spots of soft decay.
Cauliflower	White to creamy compact solid and clean curds (head). A slightly granular texture of the curd will not hurt the eating quality if the surface is compact. Ignore small green leaflets extending through the curd. If jacket leaves are attached, a green color is a sign of freshness.	A spreading of the curd—a sign of aging or over-maturity. Avoid wilting or discolored spots on the curd. A smudgy or speckled appearance of the curd is a sign of insect injury, mold growth, or decay and should be avoided.

VEGETABLE BUYING GUIDE (CONTINUED)

Vegetable	What To Look For	What To Avoid
Celery	Freshness and crispness: the stalk should have a solid, rigid feel, and leaflets should be fresh or only slightly wilted. Look for a glossy surface, light or medium green stalks, and green leaflets.	Wilted celery with flabby upper branches or leaf stems. Celery with pithy, hollow, or discolored centers in the branches. Celery with internal discoloration will show some gray or brown on the inside surface of the larger branches near the base of the stock. Avoid celery with "blackheart," a brown or black discoloration of the small center branches; insect injury in the center branches or the insides of outer branches; long, thick seedstem in place of the usually small, tender heart branches.
Chicory, Endive, Escarole	Freshness, crispness, and tenderness: look for a good green color of the outer leaves (except for Witloof or Belgian endive, the compact, cigar-shaped creamy white endive grown in complete darkness).	Plants with leaves that have brownish or yellowish discoloration or insect injury.
Chinese Cabbage	Fresh, crisp, green plants that are free from blemishes or decay.	Wilted or yellowed plants.
Corn	Fresh, succulent husks with good green color, silk ends that are free from decay or work injury, and stem ends (opposite from the silk) that are not too discolored or dried. Select ears that are well covered with plump, not-too-mature kernels.	Ears with undeveloped kernels that lack yellow color (in yellow corn), ears with very large kernels, and ears with dark yellow kernels with depressed areas on the outer surface. Avoid ears of corn with yellowed, wilted, or dried husks, or discolored and dried out stem ends.
Cucumbers	Cucumbers with good green color that are firm over their entire length. They should be well shaped and well developed, but should not be too large in diameter. Good cucumbers typically have small lumps on their surfaces. They also may have some white or greenish white color and still be of top quality.	Overgrown cucumbers that are large in diameter and have a dull color, turning yellowish. Also avoid cucumbers with withered or shriveled ends—signs of toughness and bitter flavor.
Eggplant	Firm, heavy, smooth, and uniformly dark purple eggplants.	Those that are poorly colored, soft, shriveled, cut, or that show decay in the form of irregular dark brown spots.

VEGETABLE BUYING GUIDE (CONTINUED)

Vegetable	What To Look For	What To Avoid
Greens (chard, collard, kale, mustard, turnip, spinach, beet greens)	Leaves that are fresh, young, tender, free from blemishes and that have a good, healthy green color. Beet tops and ruby chard show reddish color.	Leaves with coarse, fibrous stems, yellowish green color, softness (a sign of decay), or a wilted condition. Avoid greens with evidence of insects—especially aphids—which are sometimes hard to see and equally hard to wash away.
Lettuce	Iceberg and Romaine lettuce leaves should be crisp. Other lettuce types will have a softer texture, but leaves should not be wilted. Look for a good, bright color, medium to light green in most varieties.	Heads of iceberg that are very hard and that lack green color (signs of over-maturity). Such heads sometimes develop discoloration in the center of the leaves (the "mid-ribs"), and may have a less attractive flavor. Avoid heads with irregular shapes and hard bumps on top, which indicate the presence of overgrown central stems. Check the lettuce for tip burn, a tan or brown area (dead tissue) around the margins of the leaves. Slight discoloration of the outer or wrapper leaves usually will not hurt the quality of the lettuce but serious discoloration or soft decay definitely should be avoided.
Mushrooms	Young mushrooms that are small to medium in size. Caps should be either closed around the stem or moderately open with pink or light tan gills. The surface of the cap should be white or creamy, or from some producing areas, light brown.	Overripe mushrooms (shown by wide-open caps and dark, discolored gills underneath) and those with pitted or seriously discolored caps.
Okra	Tender pods (the tips will bend with very slight pressure) under 4½ inches (11 cm) long. They should have a bright green color and be free from blemishes.	Tough, fibrous pods, indicated by tips that are stiff and resist bending, or by a very hard body of the pod, or by pale, faded green color.
Onions (dry onions)	Hard or firm onions that are dry and have small necks. They should be covered with papery outer scales and reasonably free from green sunburn spots and other blemishes.	Onions with wet or very soft necks, which usually are immature or affected by decay. Avoid onions with thick, hollow, woody centers in the neck or with fresh sprouts or green sunburn spots.
Onions (green), shallots, scallions, leeks	Crisp, tender bunches with fresh green tops. Choose those with 2–3 inches (5–7 cm) of white above a slightly bulbed root end.	Yellowing, wilted, discolored, or decayed tops (indicating flabby, tough, or fibrous condition of the edible portions). Bruised tops will not affect the eating quality of the bulbs if the tops are removed.

VEGETABLE BUYING GUIDE (CONTINUED)

Vegetable	What To Look For	What To Avoid
Parsnips	Parsnips of small or medium width, well formed, smooth, firm, and free from serious blemishes or decay.	Large, coarse roots (which probably have woody, fibrous, or pithy centers), and badly wilted and flabby roots (which will be tough when cooked).
Peas	Young, bright green, angular pods, well filled with well-developed peas that snap readily.	Yellow or whitish color indicates over mature and tough product. Mildew, swollen or speckled pods indicate poor quality.
Peppers (sweet green, red, and yellow)	Medium to dark green color (or bright red or yellow), glossy sheen, relatively heavy weight, and firm walls or sides.	Peppers with very thin walls (shown by lightweight and flimsy sides), punctures through the walls, and peppers with soft watery spots on the sides (evidence of decay).
Potatoes	New potatoes: well shaped, firm potatoes that are free from blemishes and sunburn (a green discoloration under the skin that should be removed before consumption). Some amount of skinned surface is normal, but potatoes with large skinned and discolored areas are undesirable. General all-purpose and baking potatoes: reasonably smooth, well-shaped, firm potatoes that are free from blemishes, sunburn, and decay. These potatoes should be free from skinned surfaces.	Potatoes with large cuts or bruises (they will mean waste in peeling), those with a green color (probably caused by sunburn or exposure to light in store), and potatoes showing any signs of decay. Avoid sprouted or shriveled potatoes.
Radishes	Medium size radishes (¾ to 1⅛ inches or 2 to 3 cm in diameter) that are plump, round, firm, and of good red color.	Very large or flabby radishes (likely to have pithy centers). Avoid radishes with yellow or decayed tops.
Rhubarb	Fresh, firm rhubarb stems with a bright, glossy appearance. Stems should have a large amount of pink or red color, although many good quality stems will be predominantly light green. Be sure the stem is tender and not fibrous.	Either very slender or extremely thick stems, which are likely to be tough; also avoid wilted or flabby rhubarb.
Squash (summer)	Squash that is tender but firm, well formed and developed, fairly heavy in relation to size, and fresh appearing. The skin of a tender squash is glossy instead of dull and is neither hard nor tough. Seeds are soft and fully edible.	Over mature squash will have a dull appearance and a hard, tough surface. Such squash usually have enlarged seeds and dry stringy flesh.

VEGETABLE BUYING GUIDE (CONTINUED)

Vegetable	What To Look For	What To Avoid
Squash (fall and winter)	Full maturity, indicated by a hard, tough rind. Also look for squash that is heavy for its size (meaning a thick wall and more edible flesh).	Squash with cuts, punctures, sunken or moldy spots on the rind—all indications of decay. A tender rind indicates immaturity that is a sign of poor eating quality in winter squash varieties.
Sweet Potatoes	Well-shaped firm sweet potatoes with smooth, bright, uniformly colored skins, free from signs of decay. Because they are more perishable than white potatoes, extra care should be used in selecting sweet potatoes.	Sweet potatoes with worm holes, cuts, grub injury, or any other defects that penetrate the skin; this causes waste and can readily lead to decay. Even when the decayed portion is cut away, the remainder of the potato flesh that looks normal may have a bad taste. Decay is the worst problem with sweet potatoes and is of three types: wet, soft decay; dry, firm decay, which begins at the end of the potato, making it discolored and shriveled; and dry rot in the form of sunken, discolored areas on the sides of the potato.
Tomatoes	Tomatoes that are well formed, smooth, well-ripened, and reasonably free from blemishes. For fully ripe fruit, look for an overall rich, red color and a slight softness. Softness is easily detected by gentle handling. For tomatoes slightly less than fully ripe, look for firm texture and color ranging from pink to light red.	Overripe and bruised tomatoes (they are both soft and watery) and tomatoes with sunburn (green or yellow areas near the stem scar) and growth cracks (deep cracks around the stem scar). Avoid decayed tomatoes that will have soft, water-soaked spots, depressed areas, or surface mold.
Turnips and Rutabagas	Turnips: Small or medium size, smooth, fairly round, and firm vegetables. If sold in bunches, the tops should be fresh and should have a good green color. Rutabagas: Heavy weight for their size, generally smooth, round or moderately elongated shape. Good quality rutabagas should also be firm to the touch.	Large turnips with too many leaf scars around the top and with flabby, soft, or obvious fibrous roots. Rutabagas with hard texture, pithy, skin punctures, deep cuts, or decay.
Watercress	Watercress that is fresh, crisp, and bright-green color with rather long stems.	Bunches with yellow, wilted, bruised or decayed leaves.

TABLE 8.2

FRESH VEGETABLES COOKING TIMETABLE

Vegetable	Boiling*	Steaming*	Microwave (1000 Watts)	Other
Artichokes				
French or globe, whole	35–45 minutes	30–60 minutes	High 4–5 minutes	
Jerusalem whole	25–35 minutes	35 minutes	1 medium	Bake 30–60 minutes
Hearts	10–15 minutes	10–15 minutes		Stir-fry 10 minutes
Asparagus				
Whole or butts	10–20 minutes	8–10 minutes	Spears – High 6–9 min./lb. 500g	Stir-fry pieces 5 minutes
Tips	5–15 minutes	4–6 minutes	Cuts – High 5–7 min[†]	
Beans				
Lima/green	20–30 minutes	10–30 minutes	Green beans – High 6–10 min. per ½ lb./250 mg	
Soy, green	20–30 minutes	25–35 minutes		
Green, whole or 1" pieces	5–15 minutes	20–35 minutes		Stir-fry 3–4 minutes
French	5–15 minutes	15–25 minutes	High 5–7 min. per lb. / 500 g[†]	
Beets				
Beets	30–60 minutes	40–60 minutes	14–18 minutes	Bake 60 minutes at 350°F
Broccoli				
Heavy stalk, split	10–15 minutes	8–15 minutes	Spears–High 6–10 min. per 1½ lb./500–750 g[†]	
Flowerets	4–5 minutes	5–6 minutes	4–5 minutes	Stir-fry 3–4 minutes
Brussels sprouts				
Whole	5–15 minutes	6–12 minutes	High 7–8 min. per lb. (4 cups)/500 g (1 l)[†]	Halve, stir-fry 3–4 minutes
Cabbage				
Green Quartered	10–15 minutes	15 minutes	Green, red or savory wedges—High 7–3 min per lb./500g[†]	
Green Shredded	3–19 minutes	8–12 minutes	7–13 min. per lb./500g[†]	
Red Shredded	8–12 minutes	8–12 minutes	7–13 min. per lb./500g[†]	

FRESH VEGETABLES COOKING TIMETABLE (CONTINUED)

Vegetable	Boiling*	Steaming*	Microwave (1000 Watts)	Other
Carrots				
Young, Whole	15–20 minutes	15–20 minutes	High 8–10 min. per 12 oz./340 g[†]	Bake 30–40 minutes
Young, Sliced	10–20 minutes	15–25 minutes		Stir-fry 3–4 minutes
Mature, Whole	20–30 minutes	40–50 minutes	Cut (2″) or 10–12 med. High 6–8 min. per lb./500g[†]	60 minutes
Mature, Sliced	15–25 minutes	25–30 minutes	Slices (¼″) High 4–7 min. per lb./500g[†]	
Cauliflower				
Whole	10–15 minutes	15–20 minutes	High 6–8 min. per lb./ 500g[†]	
Flowerets	8–15 minutes	10–20 minutes	High 4–7 min. per lb./500 g[†]	
Celery				
Diced	15–18 minutes	25–30 minutes	Slices (¼″) High 5–8 min.	
Chard				
Swiss	10–20 minutes	15–25 minutes	High 5½–6½ min. per lb./500 g[†]	
Collards				
Collards	30–60 minutes		High 10–15 min. per lb./500 g[†]	
Corn				
Kernel	10–12 minutes	4–8 minutes	High 6–7 min. per lb./500 g[†]	
On cob	10–12 minutes	8–10 minutes	Husked—High 2–5 min. for ear; 4½–10 min. for 2 ears	Soak, bake 10 minutes at 350°F
Eggplant				
Sliced	10–20 minutes	15–20 minutes	High 7–10 min. per lb./500 g[†]	Bake 15–20 minutes at 425°F
Kale				
Kale	10–20 minutes		High 6–7 min. per lb./500 g[†]	

FRESH VEGETABLES COOKING TIMETABLE (CONTINUED)

Vegetable	Boiling*	Steaming*	Microwave (1000 Watts)	Other
Kohlrabi				
Slices	20–25 minutes	30 minutes	High 10–15 min. per 4–5 med. (2 lb./1 kg) [†]	
Okra				
Sliced	10–15 minutes	20 minutes	High 7–10 min. per lb./500 g[†]	
Onions				
Small Whole	15–30 minutes	25–35 minutes	High 7–10 min. (4 medium)[†]	
Large Whole	20–40 minutes	35–40 minutes		Bake 50–60 minutes
Parsnips				
Whole	20–40 minutes	30–45 minutes	High 4–6 min. per lb./500 g[†]	Bake 45–60 minutes
Quartered	5–10 minutes	8–10 minutes		
Peas				
Green	8–10 minutes	5–8 minutes	High 5–7 min. per lb. (2 cups)/500 g (500 ml) Pea Pod—High 2–4 min. 1/4 lb. /125 g[†]	
Potatoes (white)				
Medium	25–40 minutes	30–45 minutes	Baked—High 3–5 min. one med; 5–7½ min. two med[†]	Bake 45–60 minutes
Whole			Boiled whole–High 5–8 min. per eight med	
Quartered	20–25 minutes	20–30 minutes	Slices–(¼") 5–7 min. per 4 med[†]	
Rutabaga				
Diced	20–30 minutes	35–45 minutes	High 14–18 min. per 1½ lbs. (3–4 cups)/ 750 g (0.7–1 l)[†]	
Spinach				
Spinach	5–6 minutes	2–5 minutes	High 7 min. per lb./500 g[†]	

FRESH VEGETABLES COOKING TIMETABLE (CONTINUED)

Vegetable	Boiling*	Steaming*	Microwave (1000 Watts)	Other
Squash				
Hubbard 2" pieces	15–20 minutes	25–40 minutes	Winter—High 6–7 min. per lb. / 500 g†	Bake 40–60 minutes
Summer, Sliced	8–15 minutes	15–20 minutes	Summer–(¼" slices) 2½–6½ min. per 2 cups / 500 ml†	High Bake 30 minutes
Sweet Potatoes (Yams)				
Whole	30–35 minutes	35–55 minutes	High 3–5 min. per potato; 5–9 min. for two potatoes	Bake 30–45 minutes
Quartered	15–25 minutes	25–35 minutes		
Tomatoes				
Tomatoes	7–15 minutes		High 4–6 min. per lb. / 500 g†	Bake 15–30 minutes
Turnips				
Whole	20– 30 minutes		Slices (¼") High 9–11 min.	
Sliced	15–25 minutes	20–25 minutes	4 med cubes (½") High 12–14 min. per 4 med†	

* For altitude cookery, increase cooking time 4 to11% at 5,000 feet (1524 m); 20 to 25% percent at 7,200 ft (2194 m); and 55 to 66% at 10,000 feet (3048 m) and add more water.

† Rest covered 3 minutes.

TABLE 8.3

GUIDE TO HERB-VEGETABLE COOKERY

Vegetable	Appropriate Spice or Herb
Asparagus	Cayenne or red pepper, celery flakes, cinnamon, mustard seed, nutmeg, poppy seeds, sesame seed, tarragon
Lima Beans	Marjoram, oregano, rosemary, sage, savory, tarragon, thyme
Green Beans	Basil, dill, marjoram, mint, mustard seed, nutmeg, oregano, tarragon, poultry seasoning, rosemary, savory, thyme
Beets	Allspice, bay leaves, caraway seed, cloves, cinnamon, dill, ginger, mustard seed, savory, thyme
Broccoli	Caraway seed, cayenne or red pepper, celery flakes, dill, herb seasoning, lemon or orange bits, mustard seed, nutmeg, tarragon, thyme

GUIDE TO HERB-VEGETABLE COOKERY (CONTINUED)

Vegetable	Appropriate Spice or Herb
Brussels Sprouts	Basil, caraway seed, dill, mustard seed, rosemary, sage, thyme
Cabbage	Caraway seed, celery seed, dill, mint, mustard seed, nutmeg, rosemary, savory, tarragon
Carrots	Allspice, bay leaves, basil leaves, caraway seed, chili powder, fennel, cinnamon, dill, ginger, lemon or orange bits, mace, marjoram, mint, nutmeg, oregano, parsley flakes, poppy seed, pumpkin pie spice, rosemary, thyme
Cauliflower	Basil leaves, caraway seed, celery salt, dill, mace, mustard seeds, parsley flakes, rosemary, tarragon
Corn	Cayenne or red pepper, celery flakes, chili powder, mustard seeds
Cucumbers	Basil, dill, mint, tarragon
Eggplant	Allspice, cayenne or red pepper, chili powder, basil leaves, herb seasoning
Mushrooms	Herb seasoning, marjoram, sesame seed
Okra	Celery seed
Onions	Caraway seed, cayenne or red pepper, chili powder, cloves, mustard seed, nutmeg, oregano, parsley, sage flakes, poultry seasoning, thyme
Peas	Basil leaves, dill, marjoram, mint, oregano, poppy seed, rosemary, sage, savory
Potatoes	Basil leaves, bay leaves, caraway seed, celery seed, chives, dill, herb seasoning, mustard seed, oregano, parsley flakes, poppy seed, rosemary, thyme
Rutabagas	Pumpkin pie spice
Spinach	Allspice, basil leaves, mace, lemon or orange bits, marjoram, nutmeg, oregano
Squash	Allspice, basil leaves, cardamom, cinnamon, cloves, fennel, ginger, lemon or orange bits, marjoram, mustard seed, nutmeg, oregano, pumpkin pie spice, rosemary, thyme
Sweet potatoes	Allspice, cardamom, cinnamon, cloves, ginger, lemon or orange bits, nutmeg
Tomatoes	Basil, bay leaves, celery seed, cloves, herb seasoning, oregano, parsley flakes, rosemary, sage, sesame seed, tarragon, thyme
Turnips	Oregano, poppy seed, rosemary
Green salads	Basil, chives, dill, tarragon

Note: Curry powder adds piquancy to creamed vegetables. Pepper and parsley may be used with any of the vegetables.

CHAPTER 9: Grain Products

Cereal grains are the seeds of cultivated grasses, including barley, corn, oats, rice, and wheat. The kernels of the various grains are similar in structure but differ in size and shape. The three main structural parts of the kernel are bran, which is the outer protective covering of the kernel; endosperm, which comprises about 85 percent of the kernel and contains the food supply of the plant; and germ, which contains elements necessary for new plant life.

BARLEY PRODUCTS

In the United States, this grain is sold mainly as pearl barley, which is the whole grain with hull and bran removed. It is used principally as a soup ingredient. Pearl barley may be used in casseroles, pilafs, or salads. The grain also may be made into a flour by a process similar to that for making wheat flour. Barley flour and milling fractions such as bran, middlings, and shorts are used in baked products and breakfast cereals. Barley products are high in soluble fiber.

CORN PRODUCTS

Cornmeal is made by grinding white or yellow corn kernels to a fineness specified by federal standards. Corn meals contain small amounts of fat and crude fiber and not more than 15 percent moisture. De-germed cornmeal is made by grinding the kernel after the germ is removed.

Bolted white or yellow cornmeal is ground finer than the cornmeal described above but otherwise is similar.

Enriched cornmeal contains added vitamins and minerals. It is enriched with thiamin, riboflavin, niacin, and iron. It also may contain calcium and Vitamin D.

Corn flour may be a byproduct in the preparation of cornmeal or may be prepared especially by milling and sifting yellow or white corn.

Corn grits, grits, or hominy grits are made from white or yellow corn from which the bran and germ have been removed. Grits are more coarsely ground than cornmeal.

Hominy is corn with the hull and germ removed, left whole, or broken into particles. Pearl hominy is whole grain hominy with the hulls removed by machinery. Lye hominy is whole grain hominy that has been soaked in lye water to remove the hulls. Granulated hominy is a ground form of hominy. Hominy grits are broken grains.

Cornstarch is the refined starch obtained from the endosperm of corn.

Waxy cornstarch is prepared from waxy corn. It is composed almost completely of amylopectin with little or no amylose. This starch acts as a stabilizer for frozen sauces and pie fillings.

Flavored cornstarch mixes are blends of cornstarch, sugar, and flavorings for making puddings and pie fillings. Instant cornstarch puddings usually contain dehydrated gelatinized cornstarch, sugar or sugar substitute, and flavoring.

Corn cereals are usually ready-to-eat flakes or puffs made from corn grits that have been cooked and dried or toasted. Corn cereals may be flavored, sugarcoated, and enriched with thiamin, riboflavin, niacin, and iron, or fortified with vitamins and minerals.

OAT PRODUCTS

Oatmeal, or rolled oats, also called oats, is made by rolling the groats (oats with hulls removed) to form flakes. Regular oats and quick-cooking oats differ only in thinness of flakes. For quick-cooking oats, the finished groats (edible portion of the kernel) are cut into tiny particles that are then rolled into thin, small flakes. Steel-cut oats, those that are not flaked, are the most resistant of the oat products to overcooking. Although oatmeal is considered primarily a breakfast cereal, many recipes call for its use in cooking and baking.

Oat bran is essentially the envelope of the groat, composed of the outermost pericarp. Oat bran is high in soluble fiber and can be used in many types of recipes.

RICE PRODUCTS

Rice grains are classified as long grain, medium grain, and short grain, according to varieties. Both medium- and short-grain rice have a higher proportion of amylopectin than long-grain rice and therefore the grains cling together after cooking. **Brown rice** is the grain from which only the hull has been removed. It has a nutty flavor when cooked. The bran and germ are high in fiber, minerals, and vitamins. **White rice** has the bran and germ layers removed and is the starchy endosperm of the grain.

Aromatic rice has a natural aroma of florals, roasted nuts, or popcorn. Special varieties of rice are aromatic; nothing is added to the grains. Aromatic rice includes basmati, jasmine, Texmati, Wehani, and wild pecan rice. New cultivars are being developed with other aromas and flavors.

Enriched rice contains thiamin, riboflavin, niacin, folic acid, and iron. Over 90 percent of milled rice in the United States is enriched. Enriched rice should not be rinsed before or after cooking.

Imported rice includes arborio rice from Italy, which is used to make risotto, a creamy rice dish. U.S. medium- or short-grain rice may be substituted for arborio rice.

Precooked or instant rice is packaged long-grain rice (brown or white) that has been cooked, rinsed, and dried by a patented process.

Parboiled or converted rice has been steeped in warm or hot water, drained, steamed under pressure, and dried before it is hulled and milled. This steaming process causes vitamins and minerals present in the outer coats to migrate to the interior of the kernel. Parboiling gelatinizes some of the starch, which results in a shorter cooking time.

Rice bran consists of bran and germ. It is a smooth brown powder with a faintly sweet taste; it is rich in nutrients and fiber.

Rice polish consists of inner bran layers and some endosperm. It is a smooth yellow powder with a sweet taste.

Rice flour is made from white or brown rice ground into flour. It is gluten-free and can be used by those who are allergic to wheat flour.

Sweet or waxy rice flour is made from waxy rice. It is composed almost completely of amylopectin with little or no amylose. It acts as a stabilizer in sauces and gravies and is especially useful in preventing separation in these products when they are frozen.

CLASSES OF WHEAT

There are six classes of wheat grown in the United States. They are durum wheat for pasta; hard red spring, hard red winter, and hard white for yeast breads and hard rolls; soft red winter for flat breads, cakes, pastries, and crackers; soft white wheat for flat breads, cakes, pastries, crackers, and noodles.

WHEAT PRODUCTS

Bulgur wheat is whole wheat that has been cooked, dried, partly debranned, and cracked into coarse, angular fragments. Rehydration requires simmering for 15 to 25 minutes. It may be used as an alternate for rice in many recipes and resembles whole wheat in nutritional properties.

Cracked wheat is similar to bulgur in nutrition and texture but it has not been precooked. It is the whole kernel broken into smaller pieces that serves as a hot cereal or an addition to baked goods. Cracked wheat should be pre-soaked or cooked before adding it to baked products.

Farina is the coarsely ground endosperm of wheats other than durum. It is the prime ingredient in many hot breakfast cereals and is occasionally used for pasta. Enriched farina contains thiamin, riboflavin, niacin, folic acid, and iron. Calcium and Vitamin D also may be added.

Semolina is the coarsely ground endosperm of durum wheat. The primary use of semolina is for pasta; however, it is also used for couscous, a tiny rice-grain sized pasta used in Moroccan cooking.

Wheat bran is the outer layer of the kernel. It is high in insoluble fiber and can be added to baked goods, casseroles, cereals, and meat dishes.

Wheat germ is the germ of the kernel and is often added to baked goods, casseroles, and beverages to enhance the nutritional value and give a nutty, crunchy texture. Because of the oil content, it should be tightly covered and stored in the refrigerator or freezer.

Wheat kernels (berries) are the whole-grain kernel; they can be sprouted and added to salads and baked goods. The cooked berries can be used as a meat extender, breakfast cereal, or a substitute for beans in chili, salads, and baked dishes.

FLOURS

The term *flour*, when used in recipes, is understood to mean refined all-purpose wheat flour unless otherwise designated as, for example, bread flour, cake flour, self-rising flour, oat flour, or rice flour. The majority of states require white flour to be enriched. Therefore, the major mills in the United States enrich all their flour so it can be shipped interstate. The Federal standards for enriched corn, rice, macaroni, and wheat flour are presented in Table 9.1. The following describes in more detail the various types of wheat flour available in most markets.

All-purpose flour is the finely ground endosperm of the wheat kernel separated from the bran and germ during milling. It is made from hard wheats (other than durum) or a combination of hard and soft wheats. It is best for quick breads and may be used for yeast breads, cakes, pastry, and cookies.

Bread flour is the ground endosperm from hard wheats and is best for yeast breads because of its high gluten content (higher in percent and stronger in viscoelastic qualities than all-purpose flour).

Cake flour is milled from the endosperm of soft wheats and is especially suited for cakes, cookies, and crackers. Because it is so fine and uniform, it feels soft and satiny. It is low in gluten and forms a more delicate structure than all-purpose flour.

Enriched flour is white flour that contains added vitamins and minerals. Thiamin, riboflavin, niacin, folic acid, and iron are added; the addition of calcium is optional.

Gluten flour is a mixture of wheat flour and gluten with a protein content of about 45 percent vs. 13 percent for bread flour, 11 percent for all-purpose, and 8 to 9 percent for cake flour.

TABLE 9.1

FEDERAL STANDARDS FOR ENRICHED CORN, RICE, MACARONI, AND WHEAT FLOUR

Nutrient	Farina	Corn Meal	Rice	Macaroni	Wheat
Required per pound (454 g) of flour:					
Thiamin	2.0 – 2.5 mg	2.0 – 3.0 mg	2.0 – 4.0 mg	4.0 – 5.0 mg	2.9 mg
Riboflavin	1.2 – 1.5 mg	1.2 – 1.8 mg		1.7 – 2.2 mg	1.8 mg
Niacin	16 – 20 mg	16 – 24 mg	16 – 32 mg	27 – 34 mg	24 mg
Iron	13 mg	13 – 26 mg	13 – 26 mg	13 – 16.5 mg	20 mg
Folic Acid	0.7– 0.87 mg	0.7– 1.0 mg	0.7– 1.4 mg	0.9– 1.2 mg	0.7 mg
Optional per pound (454 g) of flour:					
Calcium	500 mg	500 – 750 mg		500 – 625 mg	960 mg
Vitamin D	250 IU	250 – 1000 IU		250 – 1000 mg	
Riboflavin			1.2 – 2.4 mg		

Instant, instantized, instant-blending, or quick-mixing flour is a granular all-purpose flour that blends more readily with liquids than regular flour. It is made by exposing all-purpose flour to hot water or steam to combine the individual particles into agglomerates. It is excellent for gravies and as a thickener but also can be used in baked goods with some adaptations.

Pastry flour is milled from the endosperm of soft wheats and is used in pastries.

Self-rising flour is an all-purpose flour with 1½ teaspoons (7.5 ml) of baking powder and ½ teaspoon (2.5 ml) of salt added per cup (250 ml) of flour. It can be substituted for all-purpose flour by reducing the baking powder and salt in the recipe accordingly. Self-rising flour is used primarily in the southeastern United States for biscuits, cornbread, waffles, and shortbread, using special recipes.

Vital wheat gluten (also known as powdered gluten or gluten flour) is used by bakers to enhance the gluten quality in flour or bread products containing fiber. It contains about 75 percent protein and is made by gently washing a flour-water dough, which separates the gluten portion from the starch. The protein fraction is then dried to form a powder. Very little vital wheat gluten is needed to enhance a recipe. Use 1 teaspoon (5 ml) of gluten for every 6 cups (1.4 l) of flour and add an additional 1½ teaspoons (7 ml) water.

White-wheat flour, made from hard white wheat, is becoming popular in the United States. When the whole kernel is ground, it produces a flour with the fiber and nutritional content of the darker whole-wheat flour, but with a lighter, golden color and less bitter flavor. It has excellent baking qualities but is not readily available in grocery stores.

Whole-wheat flour, also called graham flour, is coarse in texture and is ground from the entire wheat kernel. Bran inhibits the gluten development and absorbs water, giving a heavier, denser loaf of bread. Many recipes call for a mixture of whole-wheat and white flour. Whole-wheat flour contains more dietary fiber than white flour but the other nutrients are very similar to those inwhite flour.

PASTA

Pasta includes macaroni, noodles, and spaghetti in one of 150 shapes. Durum wheat is used to make semolina, which is enriched with thiamin, riboflavin, niacin, and iron; pasta dough is made from semolina and water. Noodles are made from a more finely ground semolina and have eggs added. Pasta dough is kneaded and then forced through dies to create the many different forms of pasta available. The pasta is dried by automatic dryers which remove moisture under carefully controlled conditions. Fresh pasta is available in the refrigerated section of the grocery store. Pasta should be cooked until "al dente," an Italian term meaning tender but firm. It is best to follow package directions, but keep in mind the following: use at least one quart (1 l) of water for every four ounces (115 g) of dry pasta; add pasta to boiling water; stir the pasta when adding it, when the water returns to a boil, and occasionally during cooking; drain in a colander; and undercook slightly if the pasta will be used as part of a dish that requires further cooking.

OTHER FLOURS, CEREALS, GRAINS, AND SEEDS

Amaranth is a tall, willowy plant similar in height to corn. It has a large shaggy head containing thousands of tiny seeds. The seed can be milled into whole grain flour or puffed like rice or corn.

Bean flour can be made from many types of beans including black, kidney, fava, navy, pinto, or garbanzo. It is high in both fiber and protein.

Buckwheat is neither a wheat nor a cereal grain; it is the seed from any of the Fagopyrum family of herbs. Kasha is a word commonly used to describe cooked buckwheat groats, a Russian dish. Buckwheat is ground and used for its unique flavor to replace part of the wheat flour in buckwheat pancake mixes. It has more starch and less protein than wheat.

Millet has a stronger flavor than most cereals. It can be eaten as the whole grain. Millet can be husked, soaked, boiled, and ground into meal. It can be added in bread making.

Potato flour is prepared from cooked potatoes that have been dried and ground.

Quinoa (pronounced keenwah) is a small, disk-shaped seed that can come in many colors. It is not a cereal grain; it is the fruit of an annual herb. It is in the same family as beets and spinach. Quinoa provides complete proteins and is high in iron and fiber. Quinoa should be thoroughly rinsed before cooking in order to remove the bitter saponine coating. The whole grain is cooked like rice and it can be ground into flour and used for baked goods.

Rye flour is the finely ground product obtained by sifting rye meal. It is available in three grades: white, medium, and dark. Wheat flour is the only flour containing gluten- forming proteins that are so important in baked products because they are both viscous and elastic. Rye flour produces gluten of low elasticity; often it is used with wheat flour for volume.

Sorghum is a tropical grass similar to Indian corn and has an unusual flavor that can be improved by steaming or dry heat processing. Small amounts of sorghum are sometimes added to crackers and snack foods. Sorghum also is used to make syrup.

Soy flour is highly flavored. It must be combined with wheat flour when used in baked products because it lacks gluten-forming proteins. The amount of liquid in a recipe must be increased when soy flour is substituted for part of the wheat flour. Full-fat soy flour is made by grinding soybeans that have only the hull removed. Low-fat soy flour is made from the press cake after all or nearly all of the oil is taken out of the soybeans. The soybeans may be heat treated or conditioned with steam prior to oil extraction.

Soy grits are made from coarsely ground soy press cakes and are a low-fat product.

Spelt (triticum spela) is a predecessor of wheat (triticum sativum) and has a very strong hull that is difficult to remove when milling. It is available primarily as flour but lacks the ability of wheat flour to produce a top quality loaf.

Tapioca flour is made from the root of the cassava plant. It has a mild, slightly sweet flavor and can be used as both a flour in baked products and a thickener.

Teff is the smallest grain in the world; 150 grains weigh the same as one grain of wheat. It is available as the whole grain and flour. Teff flour can be used with other flours in baked goods and as a thickener in gravy, soups, and stews.

Triticale is a hybrid cereal derived from crossing wheat and rye. It can be cooked as a whole grain, ground into flour for use in baking, or processed into cereal flakes.

Wild rice is the long brownish grain of a reed-like water plant rather than a true rice. It is hulled but not milled.

BREAKFAST CEREALS

Whole-grain cereals retain the natural proportion of bran, germ, and endosperm, and the specific nutrients that are normally contained in the whole, unprocessed grain.

Enriched cereals contain added amounts of thiamin, riboflavin, niacin, and iron. The levels of nutrient enrichment are established by FDA.

Fortified cereals contain added amounts of selected nutrients that may or may not have been present in the grain before processing.

Restored cereals contain added amounts of selected nutrients to supply the same approximate levels of these nutrients in the finished grain products as were present in the whole grain before processing.

Varieties of hot and ready-to-eat cereals include extruded, flaked, granulated, puffed, rolled, and shredded. Hot cereals include regular, quick-cooking, and instant varieties. Instant hot cereals are prepared for precooked dried grains. Disodium phosphate may be added, giving a high sodium content. The kernels may be modified with a small amount of an enzyme preparation to permit quick entry of water into the starch granules. Some ready-to- eat cereals are pre-sweetened.

STORAGE AND MEASUREMENT OF GRAINS AND CEREAL PRODUCTS

- Store flours, grains, and cereals in tightly covered containers to keep out dust, moisture, and insects; store in a dry place at room temperature. Whole grains should be stored in the refrigerator or freezer due to their oil content, which could oxidize and become rancid.

- Store dried pasta or egg noodles tightly covered or well wrapped. These products may be stored for one year. Follow package directions for storage of commercially prepared fresh pasta. Fresh pasta must be refrigerated and should be eaten within two days or frozen for later use.

- Cereals may be stored satisfactorily for two to three months; cornmeal and hominy grits for four to six months; bulgur and brown or wild rice for six months; and other rices for one year.

- To measure sifted or unsifted all-purpose flour, sift into a bowl. Spoon rounded tablespoons of the flour lightly into a fractional measuring cup until the flour overflows the cup. Level with the straight edge of a spatula or knife. Sifting flour results in consistent, accurate measures, even if presifted when produced. Although some believe air is incorporated by sifting, it is more likely that the measure of flour is slightly lower. Therefore, it is suggested in the Substitutions section that if flour is not sifted at home, 2 tablespoons should be removed from a cup measurement.

- Today most cookbooks do not call for sifting all-purpose flour before measuring. Therefore, to measure any type of flour (all-purpose, whole grain, or meals), stir the flour gently with a fork. Then spoon flour carefully into a cup, and level off with a spatula or straight edge of a knife. The cup should never be tapped or shaken. Technically, 1 cup of sifted all-purpose flour is equal to $\frac{7}{8}$ cup of unsifted flour, so some recipes may need to be adjusted accordingly.

GLUTEN-FREE BAKING

Individuals who have celiac disease have an immune reaction to gluten, a protein contained in wheat, rye, barley, and triticale grains. The only way to prevent this reaction is to avoid consuming grains and products that contain gluten.

Gluten-free flour can be made from grains such as rice, oats, corn, soy, or millet, or from starches such as tapioca or potato. Although grains such as oats and corn do not contain gluten, they may be contaminated during milling if wheat is processed at the same facility. According to FDA requirements, for a flour or product to be labeled "gluten free" it must contain < 20 ppm of gluten.

Home bakers may use various blends of flours that do not contain gluten to prepare cakes, cookies, breads, and other products. Combinations of rice flour, potato flour, corn starch, and sorghum or bean flour are common in recipes. Eggs often are added as a binder. A small amount of xanthan gum or guar gum (about ½ teaspoon per cup of flour) is typically added to gluten-free recipes to help retain moisture, provide elasticity, and stabilize baked goods. Suggestions for gluten-free flour/starch combinations can be found in many cookbooks and online sources.

Grains and grain products contain varying amounts of fiber, both insoluble and soluble. Wheat, rye, and corn are good sources of insoluble fiber; barley and oats are high in soluble fiber. Products that are whole grain contain 3 to 5 times the amount of dietary fiber contained in refined, processed products. Some examples of fiber content are given in Table 9.2:

TABLE 9.2

COMMON FOOD SOURCES OF FIBER FOUND IN GRAINS AND CEREALS

Food and Amount	Dietary Fiber (grams)
Amaranth, cooked, 1 cup	5
Barley, pearled, cooked, 1 cup	10
Buckwheat groats (Kasha), cooked, 1 cup	5
Cereal, ready-to-eat Cheerios, 1 cup	3
Cereal, ready-to-eat Raisin Bran, 1 cup	7
Cornmeal, dry, 1 cup	6
Flour, all-purpose, 1 cup	3
Flour, brown rice	6
Flour, white rice	4
Flour, whole-wheat, 1 cup	15
Macaroni, cooked, 1 cup	3
Macaroni, whole wheat, cooked, 1 cup	4
Oats, rolled, dry, 1 cup	9
Quinoa, cooked, 1 cup	5
Rice, long grain, white, cooked, 1 cup	1
Rice, long grain, brown, cooked, 1 cup	4
Spaghetti, cooked, 1 cup	2
Spaghetti, whole wheat, cooked, 1 cup	6
Spelt, cooked, 1 cup	8

CHAPTER 10: Sweetening Agents, Fats and Oils, Leavening Agents

SWEETENING AGENTS

SUGARS

The term *sugar*, when unqualified as to source, refers to refined sucrose derived from sugar beets or sugarcane. Except for source, these two sugars are the same and are 99.9 percent pure sucrose.

White Sugar

Granulated sugar is the standard product for general use, variously branded "granulated," "fine granulated," or "ultra-fine granulated." Regular granulated is suited for most uses and is less expensive than other sugars. It is available in numerous sizes and types of packages, from one-pound cartons to 100-pound bags.

Ultra-fine granulated sugar, also called super-fine or dessert granulated sugar, is fine-grained sugar designed for special use in cakes and in mixed drinks and other uses where quick creaming or rapid dissolving is desirable. It is available in one-pound cartons.

Powdered, or confectioner's sugar is granulated sugar crushed to fine powder. These are available in several degrees of fineness designated by name or number of 3s following the name. It is used in frostings and icings and for dusting on baked products. It usually contains three percent cornstarch to prevent caking when stored in a moist environment.

Special Forms of Sugar

Cut tablets are made from sugar that is molded into slabs that are cut or clipped afterward. Cut tablets of various sizes and shapes are packed in one- and two-pound cartons.

Pressed tablets are made by compressing moist, white sugar into molds to form the tablets, which are later oven-dried to produce hard, smooth tablets. Tablets of various sizes and shapes come in one- and two-pound cartons.

Cubes are granulated sugar that has been moistened with colorless syrup, molded into cubes, and then dried. Sizes range from 80 to 200 pieces to a pound. Cubes are packed in one- and two-pound cartons.

Brown Sugar

Brown sugar is a product that contains varying quantities of molasses, non-sugars (ash) naturally present in molasses, and moisture. It may be produced from the syrup remaining after the removal of commercially extractable white sugar or by the addition of refined syrups to specially graded, uniformly minute white sugar crystals. Four grades are available for food manufacturing but only two for consumer purchase. These are variously designated as "golden brown" or "light brown" and "dark" or "old-fashioned brown," indicating the color characteristic. Intensity of molasses flavor increases with color. The granulated (Brownulated®) form of brown sugar contains enough molasses to provide a flavor intensity between light and dark brown sugars; its use in baking requires adjustments in amounts of ingredients. Brown sugar imparts flavor and color to candies, condiments, baked goods, and the like. It is packed in both 14-ounce and one-pound cartons and two-pound plastic bags. Dark brown sugar is more acidic than light brown sugar, and the proportion of light to dark affects the crystallization of candies.

Other Sugars

Raw sugar, or semi-refined sugar, has gained importance because consumers are demanding "natural products." The raw sugar available at the markets is used just like brown sugar and can be used in the same food preparations. The cost of raw sugar is high and provides no significant nutritional benefits.

Turbinado sugar is a partially refined sugar similar in appearance to raw sugar, which is sold for consumption without further refining.

Blended sugar is a combination of sugar and dextrose that may be used in place of an equal quantity of sugar, although its properties are somewhat different.

Corn sugar is dextrose (glucose) obtained by treating cornstarch with acid.

Fructose (levulose) is one of two sugars (the other is glucose) that result when sucrose reacts chemically with water. It may be produced industrially by the use of an enzyme (isomerase) to change the structure of glucose to yield fructose. It is highly soluble and is approximately one and one-half times as sweet as sucrose in sugar solutions.

Maple sugar is the solid product resulting from the evaporation of maple sap or maple syrup. It consists mostly of sucrose with some invert sugar and ash.

SYRUPS

From Sugarcane

Cane syrup is the concentrated sap of sugar cane. It is made by evaporation of the juice of sugarcane or by a solution of sugar cane concrete (concentrate). The recommended maximum ash content of the unsulfured product is 4.5 percent; sulfured, 6 percent.

Molasses is the mother liquid from which raw cane sugar has crystallized. The following types are usually found:

Table molasses, which is light in color, contains a higher percentage of sugar and a smaller percentage of ash than is present in cooking molasses. It is often sold as light molasses.

Cooking (blackstrap) molasses is darker in color and has a stronger flavor than light molasses. Barbados molasses, which is specially treated cooking molasses, resembles cane syrup more than molasses in composition. It is often sold as dark molasses.

Refiners' syrup is the residual product obtained in the process of refining raw cane sugar that has been subjected to clarification and decolorization. It is a solution of sucrose and partially inverted sucrose, containing not more than 28 percent moisture. It is used extensively for flavoring corn syrup.

From Sorghum Cane

Sorghum syrup is obtained by concentration of the juice of the sugar sorghum plant. It contains not more than 30 percent water or more than 6.25 percent ash calculated on a dry basis.

From Corn

Corn syrup (unmixed) is obtained by partial hydrolysis of cornstarch, by use of acid or enzymatic catalysts, or a combination of these. The resulting liquid is neutralized, clarified, and concentrated to syrup consistency. The principal ingredients are dextrose (glucose), maltose, and dextrins. Two types are commonly marketed: light corn syrup and dark corn syrup.

Light corn syrup is corn syrup that has been clarified and decolorized. Retail products may have high fructose corn syrup (HFCS) and/or flavoring added.

Dark corn syrup is a mixture of corn syrup and refiners' syrup. It is used as table syrup and for the same purposes as light corn syrup in combinations that give a desirable darker color and distinctive flavor. Color and flavors may be added to retail products.

A third form available to food processors is high fructose corn syrup (HFCS). An enzymatic process is used to produce syrup with 42 percent, 55 percent, or 90 percent fructose. The more fructose, the sweeter the syrup will be.

From Maple Trees

Maple syrup is made by evaporation of maple sap or by solution of maple sugar. It contains not more than 35 percent water and weighs not less than 11 pounds to the gallon.

From Bees

Honey is the nectar of plants that has been gathered, modified, stored, and concentrated by honeybees. The water content of honey is limited to about 20 percent. Its principal ingredients are levulose (fructose) and dextrose (glucose). The term honey in cookery refers to honey extracted from the comb. The different flavors of honey are classified according to the plant from which the nectar is derived.

By Special Processes

Blended syrups are mixtures of different, but somewhat similar, types of syrups that are sold for table purposes. The composition of blended syrups is stated on the label.

Spray-dried syrups consist essentially of the solids of syrup that have been spray-dried.

STORAGE AND USE

To store honey and syrups, keep the unopened containers at room temperature. Once the containers have been opened, refrigerate honey and syrups to protect against mold. If crystals form, place the container in hot water.

- Store white granulated sugar, covered, in a dry place.

- If the sugar becomes lumpy, sift before measuring.

- Store brown sugar in a plastic bag in airtight container. If sugar hardens, place a piece of foil or plastic wrap directly on the sugar and set a wad of dampened paper towel on the foil. Cover container tightly. The sugar will absorb the moisture and become soft. Remove paper when it has dried out. Brown sugar may be kept in the freezer to prevent drying.

- To soften brown sugar quickly, warm in a 250°F oven (120°C) and measure as soon as the sugar becomes soft. Sugar also may be heated in an open microwavable container in the microwave unit with a second container of ½ cup (125 ml) water for 1 to 3 minutes (depending on quality and unit). It will harden again upon cooling.

- When measuring brown sugar, pack it firmly enough into the measuring cup for the sugar to retain the shape of the cup when turned out.

- Store powdered sugar in an airtight container to keep out moisture. If sugar becomes lumpy, sift before measuring.

NO-CALORIE AND LOW-CALORIE SWEETENERS

No-Calorie and Low-Calorie Sweeteners are sugar substitutes that provide sweetness but cause little change in viscosity or density of solutions and lack other functional properties of sugar. Because of the intensity of sweetness, very small amounts need to be used, and calorie contributions, even of those that are metabolized, are considered insignificant. For best flavor, several often are combined, and dextrin, lactose, or other bulking material is included in the product. Generally, a one-serving package equals the sweetness of two teaspoons sugar.

Sweeteners that have been approved by the Food and Drug Administration (FDA) or for which petitions for approval have been submitted are shown in Table 10.1.

TABLE 10.1

HIGH INTENSITY SWEETENERS

Product	Sweeteners Index (Sugar = 1)	FDA Status	Stability	Composition
Acesulfame-K (Sweet One® or Sunnet®)	200	Approved	Stable	Derivative of (potassium) acetoacetic acid
Alitame	2000	Application withdrawn	Stable	Dipeptide of D-alanine and L-aspartic acid
Aspartame (Equal® or Nutrasweet®)	180	Approved—must be labeled that it contains phenylalanine	Unstable when heated or when stored at pH extreme	Methyl ester of dipeptide of phenylalanine and aspartic acid
Cyclamate	30	Banned in U.S. in 1970	Stable	Sulfonated cyclohexylamine
Neotane	7,000–13,000	Approved	Moderately stable	L-aspartic acid , L-Phenylalanine and 2 Methyl esters (does not yield phenylalanine
Saccharin (Sweet' N Low®)	300	Approved	Stable	Benzoic sulphimide
Sucralose (Splenda®)	600	Under review	Stable	Chlorinated derivative of sucrose

RELATED PRODUCTS

Polydextrose is a condensation polymer of dextrose, containing minor amounts of bound sorbitol and citric acid. It has one calorie per gram. As a bulking agent, it gives texture and body to foods when used partially to replace sugar or fat in some foods. Because it has no sweetness, sweeteners also may be needed.

Polyols (polyhydric alcohols). Sugar alcohols, such as sorbitol, mannitol, and xylitol have limited use in foods. Although less sweet than sugar, they contribute to texture.

Tables 10.2 and 10.3 present information on Solubility of Sugar and Temperature and Tests for Syrup and Candies, respectively.

TABLE 10.2
SOLUBILITY OF SUGAR

Sugar	Temperature		Percentage of Sugar in Saturated Solution (%)	Amount Dissolved by 100 Grams of Water (g)	Dissolved by 1 Cup Water (236.6 ml) (calculated on the assumption that 1 cup sugar weighs 200g) (c)
	°F	°C			
Common Sugars					
Fructose	68	20	78.9	375.0	
Glucose	68	20	49.7	83.1	
Lactose	77	25	17.8	21.7	
Maltose	70	21	44.1	78.9	
Sucrose	32	0	64.2	179.2	2.1
	68	20	67.1	203.9	2.4
	104	40	70.4	238.1	2.8
	140	60	74.2	287.3	3.4
	176	80	78.4	362.1	4.3
	194	90	80.6	415.7	4.9
	212	100	83.0	487.2	5.8

TABLE 10.3
TEMPERATURE AND TESTS FOR SYRUP AND CANDIES

Product	Final Temperature of Syrup at Sea Level*		Test of Doneness	Description of Test
	°F	°C		
Jelly	220	104	—	Syrup runs off a cool metal spoon in drops that merge to form a sheet.
Syrup	230 to 243	110 to 112	Thread	Syrup spins in 2″ (5 cm) thread when dropped from fork or spoon.
Fondant Fudge Panocha	234 to 240	112 to 114	Soft Ball	Syrup, when dropped into very cold water, forms a soft ball that flattens on removal from water.
Caramels	244 to 248	118 to 120	Firm Ball	Syrup, when dropped into very cold water, forms a firm ball that does not flatten on removal from water.

TEMPERATURE AND TESTS FOR SYRUP AND CANDIES (CONTINUED)

Product	Final Temperature of Syrup at Sea Level*		Test of Doneness	Description of Test
	°F	°C		
Divinity Marshmallows, Popcorn Balls	250 to 266	121 to 130	Hard Ball	Syrup, when dropped into very cold water, forms a ball that is hard enough to hold its shape.
Butterscotch Taffies	270 to 290	132 to 143	Soft Crack	Syrup, when dropped into very cold water, separates into threads that are hard but not brittle.
Brittle Glacé	300 to 310	149 to 154	Hard Crack	Syrup, when dropped into very cold water, separated into threads that are hard and brittle.
Barley Sugar	320	160	Clear Liquid	The sugar liquefies.
Caramel	338	170	Brown Liquid	The liquid becomes brown.

*For each increase of 500 feet in elevation, cook the syrup to a temperature 1°F lower than temperature called for at sea level. If readings are taken in Celsius, for each 900 feet of elevation cook the syrup to a temperature 1°C lower than called for at sea level.

FATS AND OILS

Fats and oils are substances of plant and animal origin that belong to a class of chemical compounds called lipids. The terms commonly used are "fats," which are lipids that are solid at room temperature, and "oils," which are lipids that are liquid at room temperature. Most of the lipids found in foods are triglycerides, which are esters of glycerol and three fatty acids. Other lipids found in small amounts include mono- and diglycerides (esters of glycerol and one or two fatty acids, respectively), phospholipids such as lecithin, and sterols such as cholesterol. The last is synthesized only by animals.

Fatty acids are responsible for the varied characteristics of different triglycerides. Fatty acids are organic acids, generally with an even number of carbon atoms. Triglycerides, with short-chain fatty acids, are usually liquid or soft at room temperature; the triglycerides become harder as chain lengths increase. Fatty acids may be saturated (having no double bonds), monosaturated (having one double bond), or polyunsaturated (having two or more double bonds). Saturated fatty acids are harder (more likely to be solid at room temperature) than unsaturated fatty acids, which tend to be liquid at room temperature.

Many commercially available fats are made from oils by hydrogenation. Hydrogenation is the process of adding hydrogen to unsaturated fatty acids under carefully controlled conditions to reduce the number of double bonds and increase saturation. Hydrogenation results in the formation of trans fat. Regardless of source and fatty acid composition, all fats and oils provide 9 kilocalories per gram.

ANIMAL FAT SHORTENINGS

These products are made from fat extracted from animal tissue by dry or wet rendering. The fats are then deodorized and/or partially hydrogenated and plasticized.

Lard is a plastic fat extracted from hogs. It is used in refried beans, pies, and pastries.

Tallow is fat extracted from sheep or cattle. It is more saturated than lard and has a more distinctive, meaty flavor. The flavor has made this a popular frying fat for french fries. Tallow currently makes up about 17 percent of the fat and oils used in shortening manufacture.

VEGETABLE OILS

Many of the edible oils used in the American home are of vegetable origin. Vegetable oils are pressed or squeezed from the seeds or fruits of the plant under heavy pressure (a method known as expelling) or the oils are dissolved out with an organic solvent that is later evaporated off (a method called solvent extraction). The raw oils are refined, bleached, and deodorized before being packaged. Oils to be used as salad oils are winterized by exposure to low temperatures for a period of time. These oils are then filtered to remove crystallized high-melting portions of the oil so that the remainder will stay clear at refrigerator temperatures.

Soybean, cottonseed, corn, peanut, safflower, and sunflower oils are used widely. All are bland in flavor and useful in a variety of food products. Safflower and sunflower oils, however, are poor frying oils due to their high unsaturation. Of increasing popularity is canola oil, which is extracted from a variety of rape seed and was approved for food use in 1985. Canola oil has a high content of monounsaturated fatty acids. This oil is 94 percent unsaturated. Only hydrogenated canola oil is suitable for frying.

Olive Oil

This oil is pressed from fully ripe black olives. "Extra virgin" and "virgin" olive oils are obtained from the first pressings. "Extra virgin" refers to oils with low acidity. Refined olive oil is derived from additional pressings of the fruit and is then filtered through layers of felt to remove impurities. Refined olive oil is not bleached or deodorized. Olive oil is popular because of its distinctive flavor and very high composition of monounsaturated fatty acids, a health benefit.

Tropical Oils

Palm oil, palm kernel oil, and coconut oil are sometimes referred to as tropical oils. These oils are more saturated than other vegetable oils and are popular with food manufacturers because of their shelf stability.

Sesame Oil

Sesame oil ranges from a distinctively flavored straw- to amber-colored oil (found in Oriental food stores) to a more highly refined yellow product having a mild flavor (found in traditional grocery stores). The oil is usually relatively expensive and is used primarily as a condiment for flavoring rather than for cooking. Sesame oil consists primarily of polyunsaturated fatty acids.

Marine Oils

These are oils extracted from herring, menhaden, whale, and sardines. Only menhaden oil is currently approved for use in the United States. These oils are the subject of research because they are high in omega-3 fatty acids, unsaturated fatty acids linked with a decreased risk of heart disease.

HYDROGENATED ALL-VEGETABLE SHORTENINGS

Essentially these are solidified vegetable oils. Soybean oil is used primarily, but varying amounts of other oils such as corn oil, peanut oil, and cottonseed oil are used sometimes.

The vegetable oils are refined to remove free fatty acids and then bleached with absorbent materials to remove coloring materials. The purified oils are then hydrogenated and deodorized to produce a bland-flavored fat. Mono- and diglycerides are added to enhance their emulsifying capability.

SPREADS

Butter—see page 75 in Chapter 3.

Margarine is made from refined vegetable oils or a combination of animal fats and vegetable oils emulsified with cultured milk, sweet milk, nonfat dry milk solids, water, or a mixture of these. The emulsion is then cooled and kneaded by machine to produce the desired consistency. Today, almost all margarines are enriched with carotenes to enhance color. Salt and butter flavoring may be added. The law requires that margarine contain 80 percent fat unless the product is intended as a diet substitute, in which case the package must be labeled "imitation" or "diet." Ingredient labels must state the type of fat or fats used.

Regular margarine varies in hardness due to the type of oil or fat used and the amount of hydrogenation. Spreads and liquid margarines generally are higher in polyunsaturated fatty acids than regular stick margarine. Both regular and soft margarines provide 100 kilocalories per tablespoon (15 ml) and contain no cholesterol if produced from vegetable oils. Whipped margarines have added air and provide about 60 kilocalories per tablespoon (15 ml). Diet margarines contain 40 – 45 percent fat and added water; they provide 50 – 80 percent fewer calories than regular margarine. They should not be substituted in regular recipes for the 80 percent fat products.

Blends are mixtures of margarine and butter. The products offer a butter-like taste with one-third to one-sixth less cholesterol than butter.

FAT SUBSTITUTIONS

Oils may be substituted for solid shortening in batters and doughs by reducing the amount of oil 1½ tablespoons per cup (236.6 ml). However, a product made with oil will be different from one made with shortening. Pastries will be more crumbly and mealy in texture because the oil is spread homogeneously throughout the flour mixture. Cakes prepared by the creaming or traditional method are lower in volume and coarser when oil is used as a replacement for shortening. Less air is incorporated during the creaming stage of the shortening and sugars, reducing the number of air cells that expand and divide during the baking process. To use oil in a cake, the mixing can be modified to a muffin method whereby the oil is added with other liquids; egg white foam folded into the batter at the end of mixing helps to increase the volume.

Fat Substitutes

Modified foods that may be labeled light, reduced calorie, or reduced fat are available in the supermarket. The foods may be of a fat-reduced formula or contain a fat substitute that is either not metabolized or has an energy value of 4 kilocalories (17kJ) or less per gram compared to the 9 kilocalories (38 kJ) per gram for fats.

Protein-based fat substitutes such as Simplesse® are made from egg white and milk protein that have been heated and formed into tiny spheres by a process called microparticulation. This gives the creamy mouthfeel of fat to frozen products, cream cheese, cheese spreads, or yogurt.

Carbohydrate-based fat substitutes are combinations of gums and other carbohydrates such as polydextrose that act as a bulking agent. N-Oil® is made from tapioca dextrin and maltodextrins is made from hydrolyzed cornstarch. These products contribute to viscosity and impart the mouthfeel of fat. Both protein and carbohydrate substitutes have water blended in ratios that result in a final product that may range from two to four kilocalories (eight to 17 kJ) per gram.

Synthetic-based fat substitutes include triglyceride modification (sucrose polyester), polycarboxylic acid esters (trialkoxy-tricarballylate or TATCA by Best Foods), sterically hindered esters, and polyglycerines. Triglyceride modifications are composed of modified molecules of sugars linked with long-chain fatty acids. The synthetic substitutes have the look and feel of fat but the large molecules are not metabolized and, therefore, have no caloric value. Olestra® is such a product; it has been approved by the FDA for use in replacing fat in salted snack foods. Olean is made from sucrose polyester and is used in various snack chips.

STORAGE AND USE

- Store lards and home-rendered fats such as poultry fat in the refrigerator.

- Refrigerate vegetable shortenings intended for storage of several months or more. These fats, however, will keep well at room temperature for shorter periods of time.

- Keep oils capped tightly and store at room temperature. Some oils may become thick and cloudy when stored in the refrigerator due to partial solidification. Store in dark containers or in a dark storage area.

FRYING WITH FATS AND OILS

Fats and oils are used as a cooking medium for pan-frying or deep fat frying. Oils may be preferred because they generally are more stable and have a higher smoke point than solid shortenings. Some shortenings contain mono- and diglycerides that are desirable for use in cakes, but contribute a lower smoke point. The smoke point is the lowest temperature at which a continuous stream of thin, visible smoke is observed, along with a strong odor and eye irritation. The smoke is symptomatic of a rapid breakdown of the fat, resulting in off flavor to the food cooked in the fat. The smoke point of the oil/fat must be above the temperature used in food preparation. The smoke point is lowered greatly by the presence of free fatty acids.

The formation of free fatty acids and other products from fat deterioration are accelerated with exposure to light, food particles in the fat, water from the food cooked in the fat, and a wide container with a large surface area. To maintain high quality of fat or oil to be reused for deep fat frying, the oil should be strained and stored in a closed container in cool darkness. Approximately ⅕ of the fat should be replaced with new fat or oil for each use.

Fat absorption is reduced by maintaining a high enough oil cooking temperature to allow the food to cook quickly (but not brown so rapidly that the interior is undercooked). Other factors that increase fat absorption are increased amounts of fat and sugar in the batter of the product, a lower protein content of the mixture used, and greater surface area of the product.

WAYS TO MEASURE FATS AND OILS

Butter or margarine purchased in bar form need not be measured with measuring equipment. Simply keep

SMOKE POINTS OF FATS AND OILS

Lard	361to 401° F (183 to 205°C)
Vegetable Oil	441 to 450°F (227 to 232°C)
Vegetable shortenings with mono- and diglycerides	356 to 370°F (180 to 188°C)
Vegetable and animal shortenings with mono- and diglycerides	351 to 363°F (177 to 184°C)
Vegetable and animal shortenings without mono- and diglycerides	448°F (231°C)

in mind that a ¼ pound bar equals ½ cup (125 ml) or 8 tablespoons (120 ml). Two bars equal 1 cup (250 ml).

For other fats not in bar form, use standard measuring cups or spoons. Press fat firmly into the utensil until it is full. Level with the straight edge of a spatula or knife.

The water displacement method may be used if water that clings to the fat will not affect the product. Pour cold water into a liquid measuring cup up to the measure that will equal 1 cup (250 ml) when the desired amount of fat is added. For example, if ¼cup (60 ml) is needed, pour ¾ cup (175 ml) water into the measuring cup. Add enough fat to the water to make the water level rise to the mark for 1 cup (250 ml), being sure that the fat is entirely covered with water. Drain off the water.

For oils or melted fats, use a standard glass measuring cup or spoons and pour the oil or melted fat to the desired mark.

LEAVENING AGENTS

A leavening agent is a gas incorporated or formed in a batter or dough to make it rise, increase in volume or bulk, and become light and porous during preparation and subsequent heating. The amount of leavening gas in a mixture, the rate at which it is formed, and the flavors it imparts are important in establishing texture and other characteristics of leavened products. There are three principle leavening gasses:

Air

Air contributes to some of the volume of leavened products such as soufflés and pastry. Air is beaten or folded into mixtures or introduced into ingredients by beating, creaming, and sifting. It leavens by expansion during heating.

Water Vapor

Water vapor, or steam, is formed in any batter or dough as it is heated. It is the principle leavening agent in products having a high proportion of liquid to flour, such as popovers and cream puffs. To form steam before the product coagulates, or sets, a high initial temperature must be reached.

Carbon Dioxide

Carbon dioxide is a leavening agent produced in a batter or dough by chemical or biological reactions. It is produced in breads and cakes from baking soda (sodium bicarbonate) in combination with acid ingredient(s), baking powder, yeast, or other microorganisms metabolizing sugar.

Sodium Bicarbonate and Acids

Baking soda plus an acid ingredient form carbon dioxide gas, salts, and water. Common sources of acids are sour or acidified milk, buttermilk, sour cream, citrus fruit juice, vinegar, applesauce, molasses, and brown sugar. The acidity of sour milk varies with its age and degree of sourness; the acidity of molasses also varies. The acidity of corn syrup, honey, and chocolate is too low for them to be used as the only source of acid. Then baking powder is also added. When sour milk or molasses are used, the baking soda should be mixed with the dry ingredients because the reaction between baking soda and acid is immediate in a liquid medium. For proportions of baking soda and acid to use in place of baking powder, see "Substitution of Ingredients," page 39.

BAKING POWDERS

Baking powders are mixtures of dry acid or acid salts and an alkali (sodium bicarbonate) separated by an inert filler such as cornstarch or powdered calcium carbonate added to standardize and help stabilize the mixtures. According to federal standards, baking powders must liberate at least 12 percent of available carbon dioxide. Baking powders are classified according to type of acid components. Those commonly found in the supermarket for home use, such as those listed below, are SAS and low-sodium.

- **Tartrate powders**, in which the acid ingredients are potassium acid tartrate (cream of tartar) and tartaric acid. These are quick acting or single acting baking powders that form gas bubbles as soon as the batter is mixed.

- **Phosphate powders**, in which the acid ingredient is either calcium acid phosphate or sodium acid pyro-phosphate or a combination of these. Phosphate powders may be double acting, meaning some reaction occurs at room temperature and the remaining reaction occurs with heat.

- **Sodium-free powders**, or low-sodium powder, may be double acting, in which potassium bicarbonate replaces the sodium bicarbonate. Use 1½ teaspoonfuls (7 ml) for each teaspoonful of baking powder in the recipe.

- **SAS-phosphate powders**, in which the acid ingredients are sodium aluminum sulfate and calcium acid phosphate. This type is often referred to as combination or double-acting powder and may be so considered from the point of view that the acid phosphate reacts with the baking soda while the mixture is cold, whereas the sodium aluminum sulfate produces carbon dioxide when the batter is heated. This type is always available in supermarkets and is used in home baking.

Tartrate powders release essentially all of their carbon dioxide while the mixture is cold and SAS-phosphate powders release most of their carbon dioxide when heated; phosphate powders are intermediate. Different amounts of carbon dioxide are lost during mixing, depending on the type of baking powder used.

BIOLOGICAL AGENTS

Carbon dioxide is formed by the action of yeast or certain bacteria with sugar. These reactions require a fermentation, or proofing period, prior to baking in order to produce the leavening gas.

Yeast

Yeast, a microscopic, unicellular plant, under suitable conditions of temperature, nutrients, and moisture, produces carbon dioxide from simple sugars formed from starch and/or granulated sugar. Yeast is marketed in three forms, which are interchangeable:

Compressed yeast is a moist mixture of yeast and starch. The yeast is in an active state. Presence of approximately 70 percent moisture makes the product perishable; therefore, it should be refrigerated.

Active dry yeast is similar to compressed yeast except the yeast-and-filler mixture has been dried and is then packaged in granular form. It should be rehydrated before mixing with the flour in making dough.

Quick rising yeast (rapid rising or instant) is a more active strain of yeast packaged in a dried form. It does not need to be rehydrated before mixing and is, therefore, more suitable for use in a home bread machine. For a one-pound loaf, 2½ teaspoons may be better than a whole package. Up to 50 percent less rising time is needed with this yeast than with active dry yeast.

Bacteria of certain species, under suitable conditions of temperature and moisture, grow rapidly and produce gases from sugar. Salt-rising and sourdough breads are made from dough leavened in this manner. These doughs will have a distinctive taste.

Acidic (sour) doughs contain *Saccharomyces exigus* and *Saccharomyces inusitatus*. The high acidity of the dough results in the distinctive flavor of sour dough. San Francisco sourdough bread uses, in addition, *Lactobacillus sanfrancisco*, which produces lactic acid. Other breads made from sourdough include rye breads and pumpernickel.

STORAGE AND USE

- Store baking powder, baking soda, and cream of tartar tightly covered in a dry place.

- Check the label for the expiration date, and plan to use it before that date.

- Before measuring dry leavening agents, stir the product to break up any lumps. For best results, use standard measuring spoons. Be sure the spoon is dry when the product is measured.

CHAPTER 11: Miscellaneous Foods

DEFINITIONS

Bouillon

Bouillon is a clarified liquid prepared by simmering meat or poultry. Bouillon cube or powder is a dehydrated cube or powder containing hydrolyzed vegetable protein, salt, fat, dextrin, sugar, meat extract, flavorings, and coloring.

Bread crumbs

Dry breadcrumbs are those that can be rolled fine. They are used for stuffing, for buttered crumbs, and for coating foods for frying. Packaged breadcrumbs are of this type. Soft breadcrumbs are those prepared by crumbling 2- to 4-day-old bread. These are used for bread puddings, fondues, timbales, stuffing, and buttered crumbs. Croutons are dried bread cubes sold commercially. They may have a variety of herb and spice mix coatings.

Catsup

Catsup, catchup, or ketchup is prepared from concentrated tomato pulp and liquid, seasoned with onions and/or garlic, salt, vinegar, spices, and/or flavorings, and sweetened with sugar, dextrose, or corn syrup.

Chili sauce

Chili sauce is similar to catsup but contains pieces of the whole peeled tomato with seeds and more sugar and onion than does catsup.

Chocolate

Chocolate is the product resulting from the grinding of cocoa nibs (cocoa, or cacao, beans that have been roasted and shelled). Sweet chocolate (sweet chocolate coating) is chocolate mixed with sugar; it also may contain added cocoa butter and flavorings. It is used for dipping confections. Semisweet/bittersweet chocolate pieces or squares are formed from slightly sweetened chocolate. Unsweetened chocolate is the original baking or cooking chocolate with no sweeteners or flavorings added. White chocolate is milk chocolate that contains mild flavored cocoa butter (the fat of the cocoa bean), but no additional cocoa solids. White chocolate does not keep as long as the more familiar chocolates. Couverture chocolate is a high quality chocolate that contains extra cocoa butter (32–39%). This chocolate has more sheen, is firmer than other chocolate such as semisweet or unsweetened, and is used for dipping, coating, and molding. There are several ways to temper chocolate, including the following:

1. Melt chocolate in a double boiler while stirring, taking care not to allow any steam to enter melting chocolate.

2. Once fully melted with temperature over 105°F (41°C), remove from heat.

3. Add piece of unmelted chocolate, which will provide the needed seed crystals.

4. Stir until temperature enters tempering range of 88–90°F (31–32°C). Keep chocolate at this temperature until used.

Note: Tempering range varies by type of chocolate:

Dark, no milk content	Milk	White
88–90°F (31–32°C)	86–88°F (30–31°C)	80–82°F (27–28°C)

Tempered chocolate can be stored at constant cool room temperature of 60–65°F (15–18°C) for several months without getting light brown or white coating (bloom).

Cocoa

Cocoa is powdered chocolate from which a portion of the cocoa butter has been removed. Breakfast cocoa is a high-fat cocoa that must contain at least 22 percent fat. Cocoa has a medium fat content (from 10 to 21 percent cocoa fat). Dutch process cocoa can be either "breakfast cocoa" or "cocoa" which is processed with one or more alkaline materials, as permitted under government regulations. Instant cocoa is a mixture of cocoa, sugar, and an emulsifier. It can be prepared as a beverage by adding hot liquid.

Coconut

Flaked or grated coconut is coconut meat cut into uniform shreds or flakes.

Coffee

Coffee is prepared by roasting green coffee beans and then blending, and usually grinding, them. The flavor of the brewed beverage depends on the degree of roasting. In some parts of the country—notably Louisiana—coffee blended with chicory is favored. Instant coffee is prepared by freeze-drying or by various extraction, evaporation, and drying processes. Decaffeinated coffee is prepared either by steaming and soaking green coffee with a chlorinated organic solvent or by a water-soaking process.

Fruit pectin

Fruit pectin is part of the water-soluble fiber found in fruit. In the right proportion with sugar and acid, pectin forms a gel. Commercially, pectin is refined from citrus or apple pectin and marketed as liquid or powdered pectin.

Gelatin

The term gelatin usually means the granulated, unflavored, unacidulated product. Gelatin is obtained by hydrolysis of collagen in bones and good-grade skin stock. In processing, gelatin may be alkaline- or acid-extracted. Fruit-flavored gelatin is a mixture of plain gelatin, sugar or sugar substitute, fruit acids, flavors, and coloring. It is sold in packages standardized to gel 1 pint or 1 quart of liquid (500–1000 ml). For industrial use, this product is packaged in one-pound (454 g) or larger containers.

Infant foods

A wide variety of strained, junior, or chopped foods is available. Infant foods also are labeled as beginner, second food, third food, and graduates. Food is preserved in small containers, usually glass; the food is cooked cereals, strained or chopped fruits, strained or chopped vegetables, strained meats, and combinations or mixtures of these foods. In addition, frozen dinners (usually of meat, vegetable, and pasta) are available for infants, toddlers, and preschoolers.

Mayonnaise and salad dressing

Mayonnaise is a permanent emulsion of oil droplets in water, stabilized with egg yolk. It is prepared from vegetable oil, vinegar or lime or lemon juice, eggs or egg yolks, and spices. Commercial mayonnaise must contain a minimum of 65 percent vegetable oil. Salad dressings have substantially the same ingredients as those in mayonnaise, but a portion of the egg is replaced with a cooked starch paste, and the amount of oil is less than in mayonnaise. Salad dressing is 30 percent vegetable oil. Some French dressings are temporary emulsions. Other commercial French dressings are emulsified with small amounts of vegetable gums or pectins. These dressings also contain tomato paste or purée and a minimum of 35 percent vegetable oil. Low-calorie or fat-free dressings may have a fruit or vegetable base and contain water, sugar, vinegar, modified starches, spices, vegetable gums, and emulsifiers, with very little or no oil. They also may be sweetened artificially.

Mustard
A pungent condiment consisting of black and/or yellow mustard seeds pulverized and made into a paste with water and/or vinegar. The paste may then be mixed with spices, sugar, and/or salt. Ground mustard seeds are available as a dry powdered spice.

Nuts
Nuts are dry fruits that generally consist of a single kernel inside a woody shell. True nuts include filberts, hazelnuts, almonds, pecans, Brazil nuts, and black walnuts. Cashews and pistachios are nuts (seeds) that grow on small trees. Pine nuts were commonly consumed by Native Americans of the Southwest but are now available in stores. Peanuts are the pods of a vine of the pea family and are classified as a legume. Nuts are available either in the shell or shelled. Shelled nuts may be chopped, ground, blanched, halved, slivered, plain, toasted, and/or salted. Peanut butter is a spread prepared from finely ground nuts that may be blanched or unblanched. Commercially prepared peanut butter may be hydrogenated and contain salt and/or a sweetener.

Olives and olive oil
The edible fruit of the olive tree is available in cans or jars as ripe olives, green fermented or salt-cured olives, as well as oil. Both green and ripe olives are treated to remove the characteristic bitterness of the nut. Ripe olives are packed in salt with or without spices and are available pitted, unpitted, whole, sliced, or chopped. Green olives are fermented and packed in brine either whole, pitted, or pitted and stuffed with pimiento, almonds, capers, onions, or celery. Dried or salt-cured olives also are known as green or Italian olives. The U.S. grades for ripe or green olives are Grade A (Fancy), Grade B (Choice), Grade C (Standard), and Substandard. Green olives are available in the following sizes (ripe olives have a similar size range):

No. 1 (small)	128 to 140 per lb
No. 2 (medium)	106 to 127 per lb
No. 3 (large)	91 to 105 per lb
No. 4 (extra large)	76 to 90 per lb
No. 5 (mammoth)	65 to 75 per lb
No. 6 (giant)	53 to 64 per lb
No. 7 (jumbo)	46 to 52 per lb
No. 8 (colossal)	33 to 45 per lb
No. 9 (super colossal)	32 maximum

Pickles
Pickles are cucumbers, other vegetables, or fruits, prepared by fermentation or in vinegar, usually with salt, sugar, and spices added. There are three general groups: fermented (salt and dill pickles); unfermented (fresh pasteurized); and sweet, sour, and mixed pickles and relishes of various mixtures.

Pudding
Instant pudding comes in a variety of flavors. It generally contains a modified starch, milk solids, surfactants, and a variety of flavorings and colorings.

Salsa Salsa is a combination of chopped onion, cilantro, and tomato that may contain other ingredients and spices commonly served to enhance the flavor of Mexican cuisine.

Salt Salt is sodium chloride unless otherwise identified as, for example, potassium chloride. Salt (sodium chloride) is used to season and preserve foods. Sometimes spices and/or herbs or other seasonings are added as in onion, garlic, or celery salt. Salt also may be iodized. Salt is made "free flowing" by the addition of a substance (sodium silico aluminate) that prevents absorption of moisture from the air. Unrefined sea salt is packaged with yellow prussiate of soda as an anticaking agent. Pickling salt differs from common salt in that pickling salt does not contain additives that would cloud the pickle liquid. Pickling salt may be granulated or flaked. One cup (250 ml) of the granulated salt is equal to 1½ cups (375 ml) of flake salt. Rock salt is a granular salt used in salt mills and in making ice cream. Salt substitutes contain calcium, potassium, or ammonium in place of sodium.

Soups Soups may be clear or thick and may be served hot or cold. Bisque is a rich, cream soup sometimes containing shellfish. Bouillabaisse is a fish soup or stew. Bouillon or broth is a thin soup prepared by simmering meat, fish, or vegetables in water to extract their flavor. Consommé is a clarified, double strength brown broth. Chowder is a heavy, thick soup prepared from meat, poultry, fish, and/or vegetables. Fruit soups are served as a dessert. Gazpacho is a cold soup of fresh vegetables and herbs, including tomatoes. Vichyssoise is a cream stock of puréed potatoes, leeks, and chicken stock served cold.

Spices and herbs Most spices are grown in tropical climates and herbs in temperate climates. Spices and herbs are used to season food and include various plant parts that have aromatic odors and pungent flavors. They include:

Aril (a lacy layer of the nutmeg seed)	Mace
Bark	Cassia, cinnamon
Berry	Allspice, juniper, peppercorn
Bud	Capers, cloves
Flower stigma	Saffron
Fruit	Cayenne pepper, paprika
Kernels or seeds	Anise, caraway, cardamom, celery, coriander, cumin, dill, fennel, fenugreek, mustard, nutmeg, poppy, sesame
Leaves and stems	Basil, bay, chervil, celery, chives, dill weed, marjoram, mint, parsley, oregano, rosemary, sage, savory, tarragon, thyme
Root	Root Ginger, horseradish, turmeric

Tapioca

Tapioca is made from flour obtained from the cassava root and is marketed in two forms: pearl tapioca and quick-cooking tapioca. Pearl tapioca consists of small pellets that thicken and become translucent in cooking. It is made by mixing the tapioca flour with water and cooking it on heated metal surfaces just enough to form a shell on the pellets. Quick cooking tapioca consists of very fine pellets. It is made by grinding a cooked dough prepared from tapioca flour or by crushing pearl or native flake tapioca. Flavored tapioca mixes are blends of quick-cooking tapioca, cornstarch, sugar, and flavorings.

Tea

Tea is prepared from the leaves of an evergreen tree or shrub (Thea sinensis). The treatment of the leaves after they are picked produces three types of teas. Black tea is prepared by allowing dried and rolled tea leaves to ferment before they are fired. Green tea is steamed, rolled, dried, and fired without fermentation. Oolong tea has partially fermented leaves. For special teas, including herbal, the leaves are mixed with jasmine, gardenia, mint, orange, or other spices. Comfrey, as a tea, is a health hazard when taken internally because of toxic pyrrolizidine alkaloids shown to be carcinogenic in rats. Chamomile and yarrow have long been used as teas for digestive disorders. Those allergic to ragweed, asters, or chrysanthemums should drink these with caution. Sassafras has been used as a tea; it contains safrole, a volatile oil, and a hepatocarcinogen.

Textured vegetable proteins

Textured vegetable protein products are made from edible protein sources. Extruded products are colored and flavored to resemble a food such as ground beef and are most often used as extenders. Spun soy products also are colored, flavored, and shaped to resemble products such as ham, chicken cubes, beef, or bacon pieces. Frozen, canned, and dehydrated spun soy products also are available.

Vinegars

The acidity of vinegars ranges between four and six percent (40 to 60 grain). Vinegar or cider vinegar is the product made by fermenting apple juice. Malt vinegar is the product made by the alcoholic and subsequent fermentations of an infusion of barley malt or cereals whose starch has been converted by malt. Wine vinegar is the product made by the alcoholic and subsequent acetous fermentations of the juice of grapes. Spirit, distilled, or grain vinegar is made by the acetous fermentation of dilute distilled alcohol.

STORAGE AND USE

- Store nuts tightly covered in a cool, dry, dark place or in the freezer. Exposure to air, light, warmth, and moisture can cause rancidity.

- Store spices in tightly closed containers in a cool, dry place. Refrigeration or freezing extends their shelf life.

- Keep mayonnaise and salad dressings made with eggs in the refrigerator once the jar has been opened.

- Keep gelatin in unopened package until ready for use and store in a dry place.

- To substitute fresh herbs for dried, use 2 teaspoons (10 ml) minced fresh herbs for each ¼ teaspoon (1 ml) of the dried product.

- Melt chocolate for cooking purposes in small container over hot water unless recipe states otherwise. Chocolate scorches easily when exposed to direct heat. It can be melted in the microwave oven.

- Follow storage directions when provided on package labels.

CHAPTER 12: Food Buying Guides

BUYING GUIDE FOR FATS AND OILS

Food Item and Form	Market Unit		Approximate Volume per Market Price/ Approximate Number of Servings per Market Unit		Approximate Weight per Cup	
Butter (See Dairy Products)						
Oils, canola, corn, coconut, cottonseed, olive, peanut, safflower and sesame	1 qt	946 ml	4 c	946 ml	218 g	7.7 oz
Margarine	1 lb	454 g	2 c	473 ml	227 g	8.0 oz
Whipped	1 lb	454 g	3 c	710 ml	150 g	5.3 oz
Soft tub	8 oz	227 g	1 c	237 ml	227 g	8.0 oz
Imitation (40% fat)	1 lb	454 g	2 c	473 ml	232 g	8.2 oz
Hydrogenated fat	1 lb	454 g	2½ c	551 ml	204 g	7.2 oz
Lard	1 lb	454 g	2⅓ c	551 ml	204 g	7.2 oz
Beef tallow	1 lb	454 g	3¾ c	887 ml	204 g	7.2 oz
Mutton tallow					204 g	7.2 oz

BUYING GUIDE FOR POULTRY

Food Item and Form	Market Unit		Approximate Volume per Market Price/Approximate Number of Servings per Market Unit	Approximate Weight per Cup	
Chicken					
Ready-to-cook					
Broiler-fryer	1 lb	454 g	2		
Roaster	1 lb	454 g	2		
Rock Cornish Hen	1 lb	454 g	1		
Capon	1 lb	454 g	2		
Stewing					
Cooked, boned	1 lb	454 g	2		
diced			1½	139 g	4.9 oz
Canned, boned	5 oz	140 g	1½ to 2		
Duck					
Ready-to-cook	1 lb	454 g	1		
Goose					
Ready-to-cook	1 lb	454 g	1½ to 2		
Turkey					
Ready-to-cook					
bone in	1 lb	454 g	2		
boneless roast	1 lb	454 g	4		
ground	1 lb	454 g	4		
cooked, boned					
diced	5 oz	140 g	1 to 2	139 g	4.9 oz
canned, boned	5 oz	140 g	1 to 2		

*Amounts are based on three ounces of cooked poultry meat without bone per serving.

BUYING GUIDE FOR EGGS

Food Item and Form	Market Unit		Approximate Volume per Market Price/Approximate Number of Servings per Market Unit		Approximate Weight per Cup	
Eggs, whole						
Fresh	1 doz		12 eggs		244 g	8.6 oz
Jumbo, 63 g	1 doz		3 c	710 ml	244 g	8.6 oz
Extra large, 56 g	1 doz		2¾ c	651 ml	244 g	8.6 oz
Large, 50 g	1 doz		2¼ c	532 ml	244 g	8.6 oz
Medium, 44 g	1 doz		2 c	473 ml	244 g	8.6 oz
Small, 38 g	1 doz		1 ⅞ c	444 ml	244 g	8.6 oz
Frozen	1 lb	454 g	1 ⅞ c	444 ml	244 g	8.6 oz
Dried, sifted	1 lb	454 g	5⅓ c	1.3 l	82 g	2.9 oz
Whites						
Fresh	1 doz		12 whites		244 g	8.6 oz
Jumbo, 63 g	1 doz		1 ⅞ c	473 ml	244 g	8.6 oz
Extra large, 56 g	1 doz		1⅔ c	444 ml	244 g	8.6 oz
Large, 50 g	1 doz		1½ c	393 ml	244 g	8.6 oz
Medium, 44 g	1 doz		1¼ c	355 ml	244 g	8.6 oz
Small, 38 g	1 doz		1⅛ c	296 ml	244 g	8.6 oz
Frozen	1 lb	454 g	1⅞ c	444 ml	244 g	8.6 oz
Dried, sifted	1 lb	454 g	4¼ c	1.0 l	108 g	3.8 oz
Yolks						
Fresh	1 doz		12 yolks		244 g	8.6 oz
Jumbo, 63 g	1 doz		1 c	237 ml	244 g	8.6 oz
Extra large, 56 g	1 doz		⅞ c	207 ml	244 g	8.6 oz
Large, 50 g	1 doz		⅚ c	197 ml	244 g	8.6 oz
Medium, 44 g	1 doz		⅔ c	156 ml	244 g	8.6 oz
Small, 38 g	1 doz		⅝ c	148 ml	244 g	8.6 oz
Frozen	1 lb	454 g	1⅞ c	444 ml	244 g	8.6 oz
Dried, sifted	1 lb	454 g	6¾ c	1.6 l	65 g	2.3 oz
Substitutes	16 oz	454 g	2 c	473 ml	227 g	8.0 oz

BUYING GUIDE FOR FISH AND SHELLFISH

Food Item and Form	Market Unit		Approximate Volume per Market Price/ Approximate Number of Servings per Market Unit	Approximate Weight per Cup	
Fish, fresh or frozen					
Whole	1 lb	454 g	1½		
Chunks	1 lb	454 g	3		
Dressed	1 lb	454 g	2⅓		
Fillets	1 lb	454 g	3⅓		
Steaks	1 lb	454 g	3		
Cakes, frozen	1 lb	454 g	5⅓		
frozen portions					
unbreaded	1 lb	454 g	4		
breaded, fried or raw	1 lb	454 g	5⅓		
Sticks, frozen	1 lb	454 g	5⅓		
Fish, canned					
Gefilte fish	1 lb	454 g	3	162 g	5.7 oz
Mackerel	15 oz	424 g	4¼	181 g	6.4 oz
Sardines	12 oz	340 g	3¾	159 g	5.6 oz
Salmon	1 lb	454 g	4	167 g	5.9 oz
Tuna	7 oz	198 g	2	170 g	6.0 oz
Fish, cured					
Lox	1 lb	454 g	5⅓		
Salt fish	1 lb	454 g	5⅓		
Smoked fish	1 lb	454 g	3½		
Shellfish					
Clams					
in shell (hard)	1 doz		2		
in shell (soft)	1 doz		1		
shucked	1 lb	454 g	2½		
frozen, breaded, raw	1 lb	454 g	4½		
canned, minced	7.5 oz	213 g	2½	159 g	5.6 oz

BUYING GUIDE FOR FISH AND SHELLFISH (CONTINUED)

Food Item and Form	Market Unit		Approximate Volume per Market Price/ Approximate Number of Servings per Market Unit	Approximate Weight per Cup	
Shellfish (continued)					
Crabs					
in shell (Blue)	1 lb	454 g	¾		
in shell (Dungeness)	1 lb	454 g	1¼		
crab meat	1 lb	454 g	5	162 g	5.7 oz
crab cakes, frozen	1 lb	454 g	5		
crab legs and sections, frozen	1 lb	454 g	2½		
deviled, frozen	1 lb	454 g	5⅓		
crab meat, canned	6.5 oz	184 g	1¾		
Lobsters					
in shell	1 lb	454 g	1¼		
meat	1 lb	454 g	4¾	153 g	5.4 oz
spiny tails, frozen	1 lb	454 g	2⅔		
Oysters					
in shell	1 doz		2		
shucked	1 lb	454 g	2	235 g	8.3 oz
breaded, frozen	1 lb	454 g	4⅔		
canned	5 oz	142 g	1⅔	156 g	5.5 oz

BUYING GUIDE FOR FISH AND SHELLFISH (CONTINUED)

Food Item and Form	Market Unit		Approximate Volume per Market Price/ Approximate Number of Servings per Market Unit	Approximate Weight per Cup	
Scallops					
shucked	1 lb	454 g	3⅓		
breaded, frozen	1 lb	454 g	4		
Shrimp					
in shell	1 lb	454 g	2⅔		
raw, peeled	1 lb	454 g	3⅓		
cooked, peeled	1 lb	454 g	5⅓		
breaded, frozen	1 lb	454 g	4½		
canned	13.25 oz	376 g	4⅓	130 g	4.6 oz

* One serving equals three ounces (85 g) of cooked boneless fish or shellfish.

BUYING GUIDE FOR MEATS

Meat Form	Market Unit		Volume/Number Servings per Market Unit*
Fresh or Frozen			
Boneless or ground meat	1 lb	454 g	4 servings
Meat with minimum amount of bone (steaks, roasts, chops, etc.)	1 lb	454 g	2 to 3 servings
Meats with large amount of bone (shoulder cuts, short ribs, neck, etc.)	1 lb	454 g	1 to 2 servings
Cured and/or Smoked			
Ham, boneless	1 lb	454 g	4 to 5 servings
Bacon	1 lb	454 g	24 slices
Frankfurters	1 lb	454 g	8 to 10 frankfurters

* Three ounces (85 g) of cooked trimmed meat is the usual amount of one serving.

BUYING GUIDE FOR DAIRY PRODUCTS

Food Item and Form	Market Unit		Approximate Volume per Market Price/ Approximate Number of Servings per Market Unit		Approximate Weight per Cup	
Butter	1 lb	454 g	2 c	473 ml	224 g	7.9 oz
Whipped	1 lb	454 g	3 c	710 ml	152 g	5.2 oz
Cheese						
Cheddar, Swiss and all hard cheeses (natural or processed grated or chopped	1 lb	454 g	4 c	946 ml	113 g	4.0 oz
Cheddar or Swiss sliced	1 lb	454 g	8 slices			
Cottage	12 oz	340 g	1½ c	355 ml	236 g	8.3 oz
Cream	8 oz	227 g	1 c	237 ml	230 g	8.1 oz
Spread	5 oz	142 g	½ c	118 ml		
Parmesan, grated	3 oz	85 g	1 c	237 ml	92 g	3.3 oz
Cream						
Light (table)	½ pt	237 ml	1 c	237 ml	240 g	8.5 oz
Heavy						
(whipping)			1 c	237 ml	236 g	8.3 oz
(whipped)	½ pt	237 ml	2 c	473 ml		
Sour	½ pt	237 ml	1 c	237 ml	241 g	8.5 oz
Half and Half						
(cream + milk)						
sweet	1 pt	473 ml	2 c	473 ml	242 g	8.5 oz
sour	½ pt	237 ml	1 c	237 ml	242 g	8.5 oz

BUYING GUIDE FOR DAIRY PRODUCTS (CONTINUED)

Food Item and Form	Market Unit		Approximate Volume per Market Price/ Approximate Number of Servings per Market Unit		Approximate Weight per Cup	
Milk						
Whole or skim	1 qt	946 ml	4 c	946 ml	242 g	8.5 oz
Buttermilk	1 qt	946 ml	4 c	946 ml	242 g	8.5 oz
Sweetened condensed	15 oz	425 g	1⅓ c	315 ml	306 g	10.8 oz
Evaporated						
whole or skim	14.5 oz	411 g	1⅔ c	393 ml	252 g	8.9 oz
reconstructed			3⅓ c	788 ml		
Dry, nonfat	1 lb	454 g	3⅔ c	866 ml	131 g	4.6 oz
instant	9⅝ lb	4.4 kg	4 c	946 ml	75 g	2.6 oz
reconstituted			14 c	3.3 l	242 g	8.5 oz
Milk desserts						
Ice cream	1 qt	946 ml	4 c	946 ml	142 g	5.0 oz
brick, sliced	1 qt	946 ml	8 slices			
Ice milk	1 qt	946 ml	4 c	946 ml	187 g	6.6 oz
Sherbet	1 qt	946 ml	4 c	946 ml	193 g	6.8 oz
Yogurt	½ pt	237 g	1 c	237 ml	246 g	8.7 oz

BUYING GUIDE FOR CEREALS AND FLOURS

Food Item and Form	Market Unit		Approximate Volume per Market Price/ Approximate Number of Servings per Market Unit		Approximate Weight per Cup	
Cereals/Grains						
Amaranth	1 lb	454 g	2½ c	592 ml	179 g	6.3 oz
Buckwheat	1 lb	454 g	10		170 g	3.0 oz
Bulgur	1 lb	454 g	2¾ c	651 ml	162 g	5.7 oz
(cooked)			8 c	1.9 l	230 g	8.1 oz

BUYING GUIDE FOR CEREALS AND FLOURS (CONTINUED)

Food Item and Form	Market Unit		Approximate Volume per Market Price/ Approximate Number of Servings per Market Unit		Approximate Weight per Cup	
Cereals/Grains (continued)						
Chia seeds	1 lb	454 g	10		170 g	3.0 oz
Cornmeal						
white	1 lb	454 g	3½ c	828 ml	130 g	4.6 oz
yellow	1 lb	454 g	3 c	710 ml	153 g	5.4 oz
cooked			16⅔ c	3.9 l	238 g	8.4 oz
Couscous Kamut	1 lb	454 g	10		170 g	3.0 oz
Farina	1 lb	454 g	3 c	710 ml		
cooked			16⅔ c	3.9 l	238 g	8.4 oz
Hominy, whole	1 lb	454 g	2½ c	592 ml	181 g	6.4 oz
cooked			16⅔ c	3.9 l		
Grits	1 lb	454 g	3 c	710 ml	153 g	5.4 oz
cooked			10 c	2.4 l	235 g	8.3 oz
Kasha	1 lb	454 g	10		170 g	3.0 oz
Millet	1 lb	454 g	10		170 g	3.0 oz
Oats, rolled	1 lb	454 g	6¼ c	1.5 l	71 g	2.5 oz
cooked			8 c	1.9 l	241 g	8.5 oz
Quinoa, whole	14 oz	397 g	2½ c	592 ml	159 g	5.6 oz
Ready-to-eat						
flaked					31 g	1.1 oz
granulated					88 g	3.1 oz
puffed					23 g	0.8 oz
shredded					37 g	1.3 oz
Rice, brown	1 lb	454 g	2½ c	592 ml	184 g	6.5 oz
Rice, white polished						
long grain	1 lb	454 g	2½ c	592 ml	181 g	6.4 oz
medium grain	1 lb	454 g	2⅓ c	551 ml	193 g	6.8 oz
short grain	1 lb	454 g	2¼ c	532 ml	201 g	7.1 oz

BUYING GUIDE FOR CEREALS AND FLOURS (CONTINUED)

Food Item and Form	Market Unit		Approximate Volume per Market Price/ Approximate Number of Servings per Market Unit		Approximate Weight per Cup	
Cereals/Grains (continued)						
Rice, all types						
cooked	1 lb	454 g	8 c	1.9 l	170 g	6.0 oz
precooked	8 oz	227 g			184 g	6.5 oz
prepared			2 c	473 ml	164 g	5.8 oz
parboiled	14 oz	397 g	2 c	473 ml	198 g	7.0 oz
Rye+ whole, chopped and flaked	1 lb	454 g	10		170 g	3.0 oz
Soy grits, stirred low-fat	1 lb	454 g	3 c	710 ml	150 g	5.3 oz
Teff	12 oz	340 g	1⅓ c	393 ml	198 g	7.0 oz
Triticale, whole	1 lb	454 g	10		170 g	3.0 oz
Wheat germ	12 oz	340 g	3 c	710 ml	113 g	4.0 oz
Flours						
Amaranth	1 lb	454 g	4½ c	1.1 l	102 g	3.6 oz
Corn	2 lb	908 g	8 c	1.9 l	116 g	4.1 oz
Gluten	2 lb	908 g	6½ c	1.5 l		
sifted					142 g	5.0 oz
Rice	2 lb	908 g				
sifted			7 c	1.6 l	125 g	4.4 oz
stirred, spooned			5¾ c	1.3 l	159 g	5.6 oz
Rye	2 lb	908 g				
light, sifted			10 c	2.4 l	88 g	3.1 oz
dark, sifted			7 c	1.6 l	128 g	4.5 oz
Soy	2 lb	908 g				
full-fat, sifted			15 c	3.5 l	60 g	2.1 oz
low fat			11 c	2.6 l	82 g	2.9 oz
Spelt	1 lb	454 g	4¼ c	1.0 l	113 g	4.0 oz
Teff	12 oz	340 g	2⅓ c	551 ml	147 g	5.2 oz

BUYING GUIDE FOR CEREALS AND FLOURS (CONTINUED)

Food Item and Form	Market Unit		Approximate Volume per Market Price/ Approximate Number of Servings per Market Unit		Approximate Weight per Cup	
Flours (continued)						
Wheat						
all-purpose						
sifted	2 lb	908 g	8 c	1.9 l	116 g	4.1 oz
unsifted, spooned			7 c	1.6 l	125 g	4.4 oz
instant			7¼ c	1.7 l	130 g	4.6 oz
bread, sifted	2 lb	908 g	8 c	1.9 l	113 g	4.0 oz
cake, sifted	2 lb	908 g	9¼ c	2.2 l	96 g	3.4 oz
spooned			8¼ c	2.0 l	110 g	3.9 oz
pastry, sifted	2 lb	908 g	9 c	2.1 l	99 g	3.5 oz
self-rising, sifted	2 lb	908 g	8 c	1.9 l	105 g	3.7 oz
whole wheat						
stirred	2 lb	908 g	6⅔ c	1.6 l	133 g	4.7 oz
Pastas						
Macaroni						
1" pieces	1 lb	454 g	3¾ c	887 ml	123 g	4.3 oz
cooked			9 c	2.1 l	140 g	4.9 oz
Shell	1 lb	454 g	4–5 c	0.9–1.2 l	115 g	4.1 oz
cooked			9 c	2.1 l		
Noodles						
1" pieces	1 lb	454 g	6–8 c	1.4–1.9 l	73 g	2.6 oz
cooked			8 c	1.9 l		
Spaghetti						
2" pieces	1 lb	454 g	4–5 c	0.9–1.2 l	94 g	3.3 oz
cooked			9 c	2.1 l	159 g	5.6 oz
Starch						
Corn, stirred	1 lb	454 g	3½ c	828 ml	128 g	4.5 oz
Potato, stirred	1 lb	454 g	3¼ c	769 ml	142 g	5.0 oz

Flour starch wheat, maize, rice, sorghum / Root starch = tapioca, arrowroot / Fruit starch = chestnuts, bananas

BUYING GUIDE FOR FRUITS

Food Item and Form	Market Unit		Approximate Volume per Market Price/ Approximate Number of Servings per Market Unit		Approximate Weight per Cup*	
Apples						
Fresh						
whole	1 lb	454 g	3 medium			
pared and sliced			2¾ c	651 ml	122 g	4.3 oz
sauce						
sweetened (not canned)			1¾ c	414 ml	252 g	8.9 oz
Frozen						
sliced, sweetened	20 oz	567 g	2½ c	592 ml	205 g	7.2 oz
Canned						
sliced	20 oz	567 g	2½ c	592 ml	231 g	7.5 oz
juice	46 fl oz	1.4 l	4¾ c	1.1 l	249 g	8.8 oz
sauce	1 lb	454 g	1¾ c	414 ml	259 g	9.1 oz
Dried	1 lb	454 g	4⅓ c	1.0 l	104 g	3.7 oz
cooked			8 c	1.9 l	244 g	8.6 oz
Apricots						
Fresh						
whole	1 lb	454 g	8 to 12		115 g	4.1 oz
sliced or halved			2½ c	592 ml	156 g	5.5 oz
Canned						
whole (medium)	1 lb	454 g	8 to 12		225 g	7.9 oz
halved (medium)	1 lb	454 g	12 to 20 halves		217 g	7.7 oz
Dried	11 oz	312 g	2¼ c	532 ml	150 g	5.3 oz
cooked, fruit and liquid			4⅓ c	1.0 l	285 g	10.0 oz
Avocado						
Fresh	1 lb	454 g				
sliced, diced, wedges			2½ c	592 ml	142 g	5.0 oz

BUYING GUIDE FOR FRUITS (CONTINUED)

Food Item and Form	Market Unit		Approximate Volume per Market Price/ Approximate Number of Servings per Market Unit		Approximate Weight per Cup*	
Bananas						
Fresh						
whole	1 lb	454 g	3 to 4			
sliced			2 c	473 ml	142 g	5.0 oz
mashed			1⅓ c	315 ml	232 g	8.2 oz
Dried	1 lb	454 g	4½ c	1.1 l	100 g	3.5 oz
Blueberries						
Fresh	1 lb	454 g	2 c	473 ml	146 g	5.2 oz
Frozen	10 oz	284 g	1½ c	355 ml	161 g	5.7 oz
Canned	14 oz	397 g	1½ c	355 ml	170 g	6.0 oz
Cherries						
Fresh, red, pitted	1 lb	454 g	2⅓ c	551 ml	154 g	5.4 oz
Dried, red, tart, pitted						
Frozen, red, tart, pitted	20 oz	567 g	2 c	473 ml	242 g	8.5 oz
Canned, red, tart, pitted	1 lb	454 g	1½ c	355 ml	177 g	6.2 oz
Sweet, unpitted	1 lb	454 g	1¾ c	414 ml	177 g	6.2 oz
Cranberries						
Fresh						
uncooked	1 lb	454 g	4 c	946 ml	151 g	5.3 oz
sauce			4 c	946 ml	215 g	7.6 oz
Canned						
sauce	1 lb	454 g	1⅔ c	393 ml	278 g	9.8 oz
juice	1 qt	946 g	4 c	946 ml	250 g	8.8 oz
Dried						
Currants						
Dried	1 lb	454 g	3¼ c	769 ml	140 g	4.9 oz

BUYING GUIDE FOR FRUITS (CONTINUED)

Food Item and Form	Market Unit		Approximate Volume per Market Price/ Approximate Number of Servings per Market Unit		Approximate Weight per Cup*	
Dates						
Dried, whole	1 lb	454 g	60 dates			
Pitted, cut	1 lb	454 g	2½ c	592 ml	178 g	6.3 oz
Figs						
Fresh	1 lb	454 g	12 medium			
Canned	1 lb	454 g	12 to 15 figs		230 g	8.1 oz
Dried						
whole	1 lb	454 g	44 figs			
cut fine			2⅔ c	551 ml	168 g	5.9 oz
Fruit Juice						
Frozen	6 fl oz	177 ml	¾ c	177 ml		
Canned	46 fl oz	1.4 l	5¾ c	1.4 l	247 g	8.7 oz
Fruits						
Frozen, mixed	12 oz	340 g	1⅓ c	315 ml		
Canned, cocktail or salad	17 oz	482 g	2 c	473 ml	229 g	8.1 oz
Grapefruit						
Fresh	1 lb	454 g	1 medium			
sections			1 c	237 ml	194 g	6.8 oz
Frozen sections	13.5 oz	383 g	1½ c	355 ml	219 g	7.7 oz
Canned sections	16 oz	454 g	2 c	473 ml	241 g	8.5 oz
Grapes						
Fresh seeded	1 lb	454 g	2 c	473 ml	184 g	6.5 oz
Fresh seedless	1 lb	454 g	2½ c	592 ml	169 g	6.0 oz
Kiwi						
Fresh	1 lb	454 g	3 medium			
Lemons						
Fresh	3 lb	1.4 kg	1 dozen			
Juice			2 c	473 ml	247 g	8.7 oz
Frozen juice			¾ c	177 ml	283 g	10.0 oz
Canned juice			1 c	237 ml	245 g	8.6 oz

BUYING GUIDE FOR FRUITS (CONTINUED)

Food Item and Form	Market Unit		Approximate Volume per Market Price/ Approximate Number of Servings per Market Unit		Approximate Weight per Cup*	
Melons						
Fresh						
Frozen balls	12 oz	340 g	1½ c	355 ml	231 g	8.2 oz
Oranges						
Fresh	6 lb	2.7 kg	1 dozen			
diced or sectioned			12 c	2.8 l	214 g	7.5 oz
juice			4 c	946 ml	247 g	8.7 oz
Frozen juice						
reconstituted	6 fl oz	177 ml	3 c	710 ml	268 g	9.5 oz
Canned juice	46 fl oz	1.4 l	5¾ c	1.4 l	247 g	8.7 oz
Canned mandarin fruit and juice	11 oz	312 g	1¼ c	296 ml	250 g	8.8 oz
Peaches						
Fresh	1 lb	454 g	4 medium			
sliced			2 c	473 ml	177 g	6.2 oz
Frozen slices and juice	10 oz	284 g	1⅛ c	266 ml	251 g	8.8 oz
Canned						
halves	1 lb	454 g	6 to 10 halves		224 g	7.9 oz
slices	1 lb	454 g	2 c	473 ml	218 g	7.7 oz
Dried	1 lb	454 g	3 c	710 ml	160 g	5.6 oz
cooked	1 lb	454 g	6 c	1.4 l	244 g	8.6 oz
Pears						
Fresh	1 lb	454 g	4 medium			
sliced			2⅛ c	503 ml	213 g	7.5 oz
Canned halves	1 lb	454 g	6 to 10 halves		227 g	8.0 oz
Dried	1 lb	454 g	3 c	710 ml	160 g	5.6 oz

BUYING GUIDE FOR FRUITS (CONTINUED)

Food Item and Form	Market Unit		Approximate Volume per Market Price/ Approximate Number of Servings per Market Unit		Approximate Weight per Cup*	
Pineapple						
Fresh	2 lb	908 g	1 medium			
cubed			3 c	710 ml	146 g	5.2 oz
Frozen chunks	13.5 oz	383 g	1½ c	355 ml	204 g	7.2 oz
Canned						
chunks, tidbits	29 oz	822 g	3¾ c	887 ml	198 g	7.0 oz
crushed	29 oz	822 g	3¾ c	887 ml	260g	9.2 oz
sliced	20 oz	567 g	10 slices		208 g	7.3 oz
juice	46 fl oz	1.4 l	5¾ c	1.4 l		
Dried	1 lb	454 g	3 c	710 ml	160 g	5.6 oz
Plums						
Fresh	1 lb	454 g	8 to 20 plums			
halved			2 c	473 ml	185 g	6.5 oz
Canned, whole	1 lb	454 g	10 to 14 plums		223 g	7.9 oz
Prunes (dried plums)						
Canned	1 lb	454 g	10 to 14 prunes		196 g	6.9 oz
Dried						
whole	1 lb	454 g	2½ c	592 ml	176 g	6.2 oz
cooked			4–4½ c	946–1065 ml	229 g	8.1 oz
Dried						
pitted	1 lb	454 g	2½ c	532 ml	162 g	5.7 oz
cooked			4–4½ c	946–1065 ml	210 g	7.4 oz

BUYING GUIDE FOR FRUITS (CONTINUED)

Food Item and Form	Market Unit		Approximate Volume per Market Price/ Approximate Number of Servings per Market Unit		Approximate Weight per Cup*	
Raisins						
Seeded						
whole	1 lb	454 g	3¼ c	769 ml	142 g	5.0 oz
chopped			2½ c	592 ml	182 g	6.4 oz
Seedless						
whole	1 lb	454 g	2¾ c	651 ml	146 g	5.2 oz
cooked			2¾ c	651 ml	183 g	6.5 oz
chopped			2 c	473 ml	189 g	6.7 oz
Rhubarb						
Fresh	1 lb	454 g	4 to 8 pieces			
cut					122 g	4.3 oz
cooked			2 c	473 ml	242 g	8.5 oz
Frozen, sliced	12 oz	340 g	1½ c	355 ml	168 g	5.9 oz
Strawberries						
Fresh						
whole	1.5 lb	680 g	4 c	946 ml	144 g	5.1 oz
sliced			4 c	946 ml	148 g	5.2 oz
Frozen						
whole	1 lb	454 g	1⅓ c	315 ml	204 g	7.2 oz
sliced or halved	10 oz	284 g	1 c	237 ml	235 g	8.3 oz
Dried						

*Weight per cup is that of food alone without liquid, unless otherwise noted.

BUYING GUIDE FOR VEGETABLES

Food Item and Form	Market Unit		Approximate Volume per Market Price/ Approximate Number of Servings per Market Unit		Approximate Weight per Cup*	
Asparagus, spears						
Fresh	1 lb	454 g	16 to 20			
cooked			2 c	473 ml	181 g	6.4 oz
canned	15 oz	425 g	12 to 18		195 g	6.9 oz
Frozen, spears, cuts, and tips	10 oz	284 g	2 c	473 ml	181 g	6.4 oz
Artichokes/Heart						
Bottoms			5 buttons			
Canned	14 oz	397 g	1 c	237 ml	212 g	7.5 oz
Bamboo Shoots						
Canned	16 oz	454 g	1 c	237 ml	12 g	4.3 oz
Bean Sprouts						
Alfalfa, Mung	8 oz	227 g	3 c	710 ml	75 g	2.0 oz
Fresh						
Canned						
Beans, green						
Fresh	1 lb	454 g	3 c	710 ml	114 g	4.0 oz
cooked			2½ c	592 ml	125 g	4.4 oz
Frozen	9 oz	255 g	1½ c	355ml	161 g	5.7 oz
Canned	16 oz	454 g	1¾ c	414 ml	135 g	4.8 oz
Beans, kidney, pinto, red, pink, black						
Dried	1 lb	454 g	2¼ c	532 ml	187 g	6.5 oz
Canned	15–16 oz	425-454 g	2 c	473 ml	187 g	6.5 oz
Dried, cooked	1 lb	454 g	5–6 c	1.2–1.4 l	185 g	6.5 oz

BUYING GUIDE FOR VEGETABLES (CONTINUED)

Food Item and Form	Market Unit		Approximate Volume per Market Price/ Approximate Number of Servings per Market Unit		Approximate Weight per Cup*	
Beans, lima						
shelled						
Fresh	1 lb	454 g	2 c	473 ml	155 g	5.5 oz
cooked			1⅔–2 c	393–473 ml	166 g	5.9 oz
Frozen	10 oz	284 g	1¾ c	414 ml	173 g	6.1 oz
Canned	16 oz	454 g	2 c	473 ml	170 g	6.0 oz
Dried	1 lb	454 g	2½ c	592 ml	180 g	6.3 oz
cooked			5½ c	1.3 l	186 g	6.6 oz
Beans, navy and small white						
Dried	1 lb	454 g	2⅓ c	551 ml	190 g	6.7 oz
cooked	1 lb	454 g	5½ c	1.3 l	191 g	6.7 oz
Beans, soybeans						
Dried	1 lb	454 g	2 c	473 ml	210 g	7.4 oz
Beets, without tops						
Fresh	1 lb	454 g	2 c	473 ml	145 g	5.1 oz
cooked			2 c	473 ml	180 g	6.3 oz
Canned	1 lb	454 g	2 c	473 ml	167 g	5.9 oz
Beet Greens	16 oz	454 g	2 c	473 ml	227 g	8.0 oz
Broccoli						
Fresh						
cooked	1 lb	454 g	2 c	473 ml	164 g	5.8 oz
Spears, chopped						
frozen	10 oz	284 g	1½ c	355 ml	188 g	6.6 oz

BUYING GUIDE FOR VEGETABLES (CONTINUED)

Food Item and Form	Market Unit		Approximate Volume per Market Price/ Approximate Number of Servings per Market Unit		Approximate Weight per Cup*	
Brussels Sprouts						
Fresh	1 lb	454 g	4 c	946 ml	102 g	3.6 oz
cooked			2½ c	592 ml	180 g	6.4 oz
Frozen	10 oz	284 g	18–24 sprouts			
	16 oz	454 g				
	20 oz	567 g				
Cabbage						
Fresh	1 lb	454 g				
shredded			3½–4½ c	0.8–1.1 l	80 g	2.8 oz
cooked			2 c	473 ml	146 g	5.2 oz
Cabbage, chinese	1 lb	454 g	2 c	473 ml	146 g	5.2 oz
Cabbage, napa, savory, red						
Fresh	1 lb	454 g				
shredded			3½–4½ c	0.8–1.1 l	80 g	2.8 oz
cooked			2 c	473 ml	146 g	5.2 oz
Carrots, without tops						
Fresh	1 lb	454 g	3 c	710 ml	130 g	4.6 oz
shredded			2½ c	592 ml	112 g	4.0 oz
diced					137 g	4.8 oz
cooked			2–2½ c	473–592 ml	160 g	5.6 oz
Frozen	1 lb	454 g				
cooked			2½ c	592 ml	165 g	5.8 oz
Canned	16 oz	454 g	2 c	473 ml	159 g	5.6 oz

BUYING GUIDE FOR VEGETABLES (CONTINUED)

Food Item and Form	Market Unit		Approximate Volume per Market Price/ Approximate Number of Servings per Market Unit		Approximate Weight per Cup*	
Cauliflower						
Fresh	1 lb	454 g	1½ c	355 ml	104 g	3.7 oz
cooked			1½ c	355 ml	125 g	4.4 oz
Frozen	10 oz	284 g	2 c	473 ml	152 g	5.4 oz
cooked			1½ c	355 ml	179 g	6.3 oz
Celery						
Fresh	1 lb	454 g	2 bunches		121 g	4.3 oz
Stalk	1 stalk		1 c	237 ml	150 g	5.3 oz
cooked			2–2½ c	473–592 ml	153 g	5.4 oz
Corn						
Fresh ears	1 dozen					
cooked			5–6 c	1.2–1.4 l	165 g	5.8 oz
Frozen	10 oz	284 g	1¾ c	414 ml	135 g	4.8 oz
cut kernels	1 ear		½ c	118 ml	82 g	2.9 oz
cooked			1½–2 c	355–473 ml	182 g	6.4 oz
Canned						
cream style	16 oz	454 g	2 c	473 ml	249 g	8.8 oz
whole kernel	16 oz	454 g	2 c	473 ml	170 g	6.0 oz
Eggplant fresh	1 lb	454 g				
diced			2½ c	592 ml	99 g	3.5 oz
cooked			2½ c	592 ml	213 g	7.5 oz
Greens fresh	1 lb	454 g			77 g	2.7 oz
cooked			3 c	710 ml	190 g	6.7 oz
frozen	10 oz	284 g	1½–2 c	355–473 ml	187 g	6.6 g
	16 oz	454 g				

BUYING GUIDE FOR VEGETABLES (CONTINUED)

Food Item and Form	Market Unit		Approximate Volume per Market Price/ Approximate Number of Servings per Market Unit		Approximate Weight per Cup*	
Juice						
Tomato	46 oz	1.4 kg	5¾ c	1.4 l	265 g	9.3 oz
Mixed vegetable	46 oz	1.4 kg	5¾ c	1.4 l	265 g	9.3 oz
Kolhrabi						
Fresh, raw	1 lb	454 g	1½ c slices	355 ml	140 g	4.9 oz
Lentils, dried	1 lb	454 g	2¼ c	532 ml	191 g	6.7 oz
cooked			5 c	1.2 l	202 g	7.1 oz
Lettuce						
Head	1 lb	454 g	6¼ c	1.5 l		
Leaf	1 lb	454 g	6¼ c	1.5 l		
Romaine	1 lb	454 g	6 c	1.4 l		
Endive	1 lb	454 g	4¼ c	1.0 l		
Mixed Vegetables						
Frozen	10 oz	284 g	2 c	473 ml	182 g	6.4 oz
	16 oz	454 g				
	32 oz	908 g				
Canned	16 oz	454 g	2 c	473 ml	179 g	6.3 oz
Mushrooms						
Fresh, sliced	1 lb	454 g	2–3 c	473–710 ml	68 g	2.4 oz
Canned	4 oz	113 g	⅔ c	156 ml	161 g	5.7 oz
Dried	8 oz	85 g	4 c		22 g	2 oz
Okra						
Fresh, cooked	1 lb	454 g	2¼ c	532 ml	177 g	6.2 oz
Frozen	10 oz	284 g	1¼ c	296 ml	209 g	7.4 oz
Canned	14½ oz	411 g	1¾ c	414 ml	171 g	6.0 oz

BUYING GUIDE FOR VEGETABLES (CONTINUED)

Food Item and Form	Market Unit		Approximate Volume per Market Price/ Approximate Number of Servings per Market Unit		Approximate Weight per Cup*	
Onions						
Fresh	1 lb	454 g	3 large			
chopped			2–2½ c	473–592 ml	135 g	4.8 oz
Cooked					197 g	6.9 oz
Frozen, chopped	12 oz	340 g	3 c	710 ml		
Canned	16–17 oz	454–482 g	2 c	473 ml		
Dried					64 g	2.3 oz
Parsnips						
Fresh	1 lb	454 g	4 medium			
cooked			2 c	473 ml	211 g	7.4 oz
Peas, green						
Fresh, in pod	1 lb	454 g				
shelled			1 c	237 ml	138 g	4.9 oz
cooked			1 c	237 ml	163 g	5.7 oz
Frozen	10 oz	284 g	2 c	473 ml	156 g	5.5 oz
cooked			2 c	473 ml	167 g	5.9 oz
Canned	17 oz	482 g	2 c	473 ml	168 g	5.9 oz
Dried, split	1 lb	454 g	2¼ c	532 ml	200 g	7.1 oz
cooked			5 c	1.2 l	194 g	6.8 oz
Peas, black-eyed						
Fresh	1 lb	454 g			144 g	5.1 oz
cooked			2⅓ c	551 ml	162 g	5.7 oz
Frozen, cooked	16 oz	454 g	1½ c	355 ml	171 g	6.0 oz
Canned	15 oz	425 g	2 c	473 ml	205 g	7.2 oz
Dried, split	1 lb	454 g			200 g	7.1 oz
cooked					248 g	8.7 oz

BUYING GUIDE FOR VEGETABLES (CONTINUED)

Food Item and Form	Market Unit		Approximate Volume per Market Price/ Approximate Number of Servings per Market Unit		Approximate Weight per Cup*	
Peppers, sweet, bell, green, orange, purple, red, yellow						
Fresh	1 lb	454 g	3 medium			
strips			3½ c	828 ml	114 g	4.0 oz
diced			3 c	710 ml	126 g	4.4 oz
Cooked strips			2½–3 c	592–710 ml	138 g	4.8 oz
Poi	1 lb	454 g	1 c	237 ml	240 g	8.4 oz
Potatoes, white						
Fresh	1 lb	454 g	3 medium		164 g	5.8 oz
cooked, diced or sliced			2¼ c	532 ml	163 g	5.7 oz
mashed			1¾ c	414 ml	207 g	7.3 oz
Frozen, french fried or puffs	20 oz	567 g	4½ c	1.1 l	113 g	4.0 oz
	32 oz	908 g	8 c	1.9 l	113 g	4.0 oz
Canned, whole	15–16 oz	425–454 g	8–12 c	1.9–2.8 l	179 g	6.3 oz
Dried, flakes	6–7 oz	170–198 g	4½ c	1.1 l	36 g	1.3 oz
reconstituted			10¾ c	2.5 l	212 g	7.5 oz
Dried granules	1 lb	454 g	2¼ c	532 ml	201 g	7.1 oz
reconstituted			10½ c	2.5 l	212 g	7.5 oz
Hash browns						
frozen	10 oz	284 g	4 c	946 ml	114 g	4.0 oz
	32 oz	908 g	8 c	1.9 l	114 g	4.0 oz
Pumpkin						
Fresh						
cooked, mashed	1 lb	454 g	1 c	237 ml	247 g	8.7 oz
Canned	16 oz	454 g	2 c	473 ml	244 g	8.6 oz
	29 oz	822 g	3 c	710 ml	244 g	8.6 oz

BUYING GUIDE FOR VEGETABLES (CONTINUED)

Food Item and Form	Market Unit		Approximate Volume per Market Price/ Approximate Number of Servings per Market Unit		Approximate Weight per Cup*	
Radishes						
sliced	6 oz	170 g	1¼ c	296 ml		
Rutabaga						
Fresh						
cubed	1 lb	454 g	2½ c	592 ml	139 g	4.9 oz
cooked			2 c	473 ml	163 g	5.7 oz
Sauerkraut						
Canned	16 oz	454 g	3 c	710 ml	188 g	6.6 oz
	29 oz	822 g	5½ c	1.3 l	188 g	6.6 oz
Spinach						
Fresh	1 lb	454 g	3 c	710 ml	54 g	1.9 oz
cooked			1 c	237 ml	200 g	7.1 oz
Frozen	10 oz	284 g	1½ c	355 ml	190 g	6.7 oz
Canned	15 oz	425 g	2 c	473 ml	221 g	7.8 oz
Squash, winter						
Fresh	1 lb	454 g				
cooked, mashed			1 c	237 ml	244 g	8.6 oz
Frozen	12 oz	340 g	1½ c	355 ml	242 g	8.5 oz
Canned, drained						
solids	16 oz	454 g	1¾–2 c	414–473 ml		
Squash, summer						
Fresh	1 lb	454 g			136 g	4.8 oz
cooked, mashed			1⅔ c	393 ml	238 g	8.4 oz
Frozen	10 oz	284 g	1½ c	355 ml	211 g	7.4 oz
Canned	1 lb	454 g				

BUYING GUIDE FOR VEGETABLES (CONTINUED)

Food Item and Form	Market Unit		Approximate Volume per Market Price/ Approximate Number of Servings per Market Unit		Approximate Weight per Cup*	
Sweet potatoes/Yams						
Fresh	1 lb	454 g	3 medium			
cooked, sliced					232 g	8.2 oz
Frozen	12 oz	340 g	3–4		200 g	7.1 oz
Canned	16 oz	454 g	1¾–2 c	414–473 ml	220 g	7.8 oz
	29 oz	822 g	3½ c	828 ml	220 g	7.8 oz
Dried, flakes	1 lb	454 g			115 g	4.1 oz
reconstituted					255 g	9.0 oz
Tomatoes						
Fresh	1 lb	454 g	3–4 small		162 g	5.7 oz
cooked			1½ c	355 ml		
Canned, whole	16 oz	454 g	2 c	473 ml	238 g	8.4 oz
	28 oz	794 g	3½ c	828 ml	238 g	8.4 oz
Sauce	8 oz	227 g	1 c	237 ml	258 g	9.1 oz
	16 oz	454 g	2 c	473 ml	258 g	9.1 oz
Turnips						
Fresh	1 lb	454 g	3 medium		134 g	4.7 oz
cooked			2 c	473 ml	196 g	6.9 oz

*Weight per cup is that of food alone without liquid, unless otherwise noted.

BUYING GUIDE FOR SPICES AND HERBS

Food Item and Form	Market Unit		Approximate Volume per Market Price/ Approximate Number of Servings per Market Unit		Approximate Weight per Cup	
Allspice	1.1 oz	31 g	1½ T	22 ml	96 g	3.4 oz
Anise	0.7 oz	20 g	3 T	45 ml	108 g	3.8 oz
Basil					71 g	2.5 oz
Bay Laurel	0.1 oz	3 g			28 g	1.0 oz
Caraway					108 g	3.8 oz
Cardamom					94 g	3.3 oz
Cayenne Pepper, ground	2 oz	57 g	½ c	118 ml	85 g	3.0 oz
Celery Seed	1.6 oz	45 g	7 T	105 ml	105 g	3.7 oz
Chervil					28 g	1.0 oz
Chili Powder	1.5 oz	42 g	5 T	75 ml	119 g	4.2 oz
Cinnamon, ground	1.6 oz	45 g	6 T	90 ml	108 g	3.8 oz
Clove, ground	1.4 oz	40 g	5 T	75 ml	105 g	3.7 oz
Coriander Seed, ground	1.7 oz	48 g	9 T	135 ml	79 g	2.8 oz
Cumin Seed	1.4 oz	40 g	6 T	90 ml	96 g	3.4 oz
Dill Seed	1.6 oz	45 g	7 T	105 ml	105 g	3.7 oz
Fennel	1.8 oz	51 g	9 T	135 ml	94 g	3.3 oz
Ginger					85 g	3.0 oz
Mace, ground					85 g	3.0 oz
Marjoram, ground	0.9 oz	26 g			28 g	1.0 oz
Mustard Seed	2.4 oz	68 g	6 T	90 ml	179 g	6.3 oz
Nutmeg, ground	1.3 oz	37 g	6 T	90 ml	110 g	3.9 oz
Oregano, ground	1 oz	28 g	6 T	90 ml	71 g	2.5 oz
Paprika	1.4 oz	40 g	5 T	75 ml	110 g	3.9 oz
Parsley	0.2 oz	6 g	5 T	75 ml	20 g	0.7 oz
Pepper, black	4 oz	113 g	1 c	237 ml	102 g	3.6 oz
Poppy Seed	1 oz	28 g	3 T	45 ml	142 g	5.0 oz
Rosemary	0.2 oz	6 g	2 T	30 ml	54 g	1.9 oz
Saffron	0.05 oz	1 g	2 T	30 ml	34 g	1.2 oz
Sage, ground	0.4 oz	11 g	6 T	90 ml	31 g	1.1 oz

BUYING GUIDE FOR SPICES AND HERBS (CONTINUED)

Food Item and Form	Market Unit		Approximate Volume per Market Price/ Approximate Number of Servings per Market Unit		Approximate Weight per Cup	
Savory, ground					71 g	2.5 oz
Sesame Seed	2.1 oz	60 g	7 T	105 ml	128 g	4.5 oz
Tarragon					76 g	2.7 oz
Thyme, ground	0.9 oz	26 g	6 T	90 ml	68 g	2.4 oz
Turmeric	0.7 oz	20 g	3 T	45 ml	108 g	3.8 oz

BUYING GUIDE FOR SWEETENING AGENTS

Food Item and Form	Market Unit		Approximate Volume per Market Price/ Approximate Number of Servings per Market Unit		Approximate Weight per Cup	
Sugar						
Brown, packed						
light	1 lb	454 g	2¼ c	532 ml	201 g	7.1 oz
dark	1 lb	454 g	2¼ c	532 ml	201 g	7.1 oz
granulated	1 lb	454 g	3 c	710 ml	153 g	5.4 oz
Cane or beet						
granulated	5 lb	2.3 kg	11¼ c	2.7 l	201 g	7.1 oz
ultrafine	2 lb	908 g	4⅔ c	1.1 l	196 g	6.9 oz
confectioner's						
unsifted	1 lb	454 g	3–4 c	710-946 ml	122 g	4.3 oz
sifted			4½ c	1.1 l	96 g	3.4 oz
Corn Syrup						
Light, dark	16 fl oz	473 ml	2 c	473 ml	329 g	11.6 oz
Honey	1 lb	454 g	1⅓ c	315 ml	332 g	11.7 oz

BUYING GUIDE FOR SWEETENING AGENTS (CONTINUED)

Food Item and Form	Market Unit		Approximate Volume per Market Price/ Approximate Number of Servings per Market Unit		Approximate Weight per Cup	
Maple Syrup	12 fl oz	355 ml	1½ c	355 ml	312 g	11.0 oz
Molasses						
Cane	12 fl oz	355 ml	1½ c	355 ml	309 g	10.9 oz
Sorghum	1 lb	454 g	1⅓ c	315 ml	329 g	11.6 oz
Sugar						
Fructose	5.3 oz	150 g	50 packets		194 g	6.8 oz
	10.0 oz	284 g	2 c	473 ml		
High Intensity Sweeteners						
Saccharin*	3.5 oz	99 g	1 g packets		142 g	5.0 oz
	2.8 oz	80 g	1 g packets		29 g	1.0 oz
Aspartame	7 oz	198 g	1 g packets		159 g	5.6 oz
	2 oz	56.7 g	2⅜ c	557 ml		
Acesulfame						
Potassium	1.75 oz	50 g	1 g packets		144 g	5.1 oz
Splenda						
Stevia						
Sun Crystal						
Xylitol						

*Brands of saccharin sweeteners vary in weight per cup.

BUYING GUIDE FOR LEAVENING AGENTS

Food Item and Form	Market Unit		Approximate Volume per Market Price/ Approximate Number of Servings per Market Unit		Approximate Weight in Grams	
					per tsp	per Tbsp
Baking powder						
SAS-Phosphate	14 oz	397 g	2½ c	592 ml	3.8 g	11.4 g
Low sodium or sodium-free	8 oz	227 g	1⅓ c	315 ml	3.5 g	10.5 g
Baking soda	1 lb	454 g	2⅓ c	551 ml	4.0 g	12.2 g
Cream of tartar	1.75 oz	50 g	5¼ Tbsp	79 ml	3.1 g	9.4 g
Yeast						
Active dry, quick	0.25 oz	7 g	1 Tbsp	15 ml	2.3 g	7.0 g
Compressed	0.60 oz	17 g	4 Tbsp	20 ml	4.2 g	12.8 g

BUYING GUIDE FOR MISCELLANEOUS FOODS

Food Item and Form	Market Unit[1]		Approximate Volume per Market Price/ Approximate Number of Servings per Market Unit		Approximate Weight per Cup	
Bouillon						
cube	3.25 oz	92 g	25 cubes			
powder	6.25 oz	177 g			177 g	6.25 oz
Bread						
Sliced	1 lb	454 g	12–16 slices			
crumbs						
soft			10 c	2.4 l	45 g	1.6 oz
dry	10 oz	283 g	2¾ c	651 ml	102 g	3.6 oz
Croutons, cubed	6 oz	170 g			51 g	1.8 oz
Catsup, tomato	14 oz	397 g	1½ c	355 ml	272 g	9.6 oz

BUYING GUIDE FOR MISCELLANEOUS FOODS (CONTINUED)

Food Item and Form	Market Unit[1]		Approximate Volume per Market Price/ Approximate Number of Servings per Market Unit		Approximate Weight per Cup	
Chocolate						
Bitter/semisweet						
chips	8 oz	227 g	1 c	237 ml	224 g	7.9 oz
	12 oz	340 g	2 c	473 ml	196 g	6.9 oz
Dark chocolate						
baking chocolate	17.6 oz	500 g	38.49		34.8 g	
Prepared drink			30 c	7.1 l		
Cocoa	8 oz	227 g	2 c	473 ml	113 g	4.0 oz
Prepared drink			50 c	11.8 l		
Instant	8 oz	227 g	1⅔ c	393 ml	139 g	4.9 oz
prepared drink			28 c	6.6 l		
Coconut						
Long thread	1 lb	454 g	5⅔ c	1.3 l	79 g	2.8 oz
canned, moist	1 lb	454 g	5 c	1.2 l	85 g	3.0 oz
Flake	1 lb	454 g	5⅔ c	1.3 l	79 g	2.8 oz
Coffee	1 lb	454 g	5 c	1.2 l	85 g	3.0 oz
Brewed			40–50 c	9.5–11.8 l		
Instant	2 oz	57 g	1¼–1½ c	296–355 ml	40 g	1.4 oz
brewed			60 c	14 l		
Freeze-dried	4 oz	113 g	2 c	473 ml	54 g	1.9 oz
beverage	10 oz	284 g	40 tsp	200 ml		

BUYING GUIDE FOR MISCELLANEOUS FOODS (CONTINUED)

Food Item and Form	Market Unit[1]		Approximate Volume per Market Price/ Approximate Number of Servings per Market Unit		Approximate Weight per Cup	
Crackers						
Graham	1 lb	454 g	66			
crumbs			4⅓ c	1.0 l	85 g	3.0 oz
Soda	1 lb	454 g	82			
crumbs			7 c	1.6 l		
fine	10 oz	284 g	4 c	946 ml	71 g	2.5 oz
Saltines	1 lb	454 g	130–140			
Wheat	1 lb	454 g	130–140			
Gelatin						
Granulated						
unflavored	1 oz	28 g	¼ c	59 ml	150 g	5.3 oz
flavored	3 oz	85 g	7 Tbsp	105 ml	179 g	6.3 oz
prepared			2 c	473 ml	269 g	9.5 oz
Infant foods						
Strained and junior (chopped)	3.25–3.5 oz	92–99 g	6 Tbsp	90 ml		
	4.25–4.75 oz	120–135 g	9 Tbsp	135 ml		
	7.5–8 oz	213–284 g	15 Tbsp	225 ml		
Juice	4 fl oz	118 ml	½ c	118 ml		
Mayonnaise	1 pt	473 ml			244 g	8.6 oz
Nuts, shelled						
Almonds						
blanched	1 lb	454 g	3 c	710 ml	153 g	5.4 oz
Filberts						
whole	1 lb	454 g	3½ c	828 ml	133 g	4.7 oz
Peanuts	1 lb	454 g	3 c	710 ml	144 g	5.1 oz
Pecans						
halved	1 lb	454 g	4 c	946 ml	108 g	3.8 oz
chopped	1 lb	454 g	3½–4 c	828–946 ml	119 g	4.2 oz

BUYING GUIDE FOR MISCELLANEOUS FOODS (CONTINUED)

Food Item and Form	Market Unit[1]		Approximate Volume per Market Price/ Approximate Number of Servings per Market Unit		Approximate Weight per Cup	
Nuts, shelled (continued)						
Pistachio	1 lb	454 g	3¼-4 c	769–946 ml	125 g	4.4 oz
Walnuts						
Persian, English						
halved	1 lb	454 g	3½ c	828 ml	99 g	3.5 oz
chopped	1 lb	454 g	3½ c	828 ml	119 g	4.2 oz
Paste, almond	8 oz	227 g				
Peanut butter	18 oz	510 g	2 c	473 ml	252 g	8.9 oz
Pudding						
instant mix	6 oz	170 g	13 Tbsp	195 ml	210 g	7.4 oz
Salad dressing						
French	1 pt	473 ml	2 c	473 ml	249 g	8.8 oz
Salt						
free-running	1 lb	454 g	1½ c	355 ml	289 g	10.2 oz
Soup						
Frozen						
condensed	10-10.5 oz	284–298 g	1-1½ c	237-355 ml		
Ready-to-serve	15 oz	425 g	1½-2 c	355-473 ml		
Canned						
condensed	10.5-11.5 oz	298–326 g	1¼ c	296 ml		
prepared			2½ c	591 ml		
ready-to-serve	8 oz	227 g	1 c	237 ml	227 g	8.0 oz
Dried	2.75 oz	78 g				
reconstituted			3 c	710 ml	232 g	8.2 oz
Tapioca						
Quick cooking	8 oz	227 g	1½ c	355 ml	153 g	5.4 oz

BUYING GUIDE FOR MISCELLANEOUS FOODS (CONTINUED)

Food Item and Form	Market Unit[1]		Approximate Volume per Market Price/ Approximate Number of Servings per Market Unit		Approximate Weight per Cup	
Tea, leaves	1 lb	454 g	6⅓ c	1.5 l	71 g	2.5 oz
Brewed			300 c	71 l		
Instant	1.5 oz	42 g	1¼ c	296 ml	71 g	2.5 oz
brewed			64 c	15 l		
Herbal	2 oz	57 g	24 bags			
Water					237 g	8.4 oz
Whipped toppings						
Dry mix	1.3 oz	37 g	6 Tbsp	90 ml	108 g	3.8 oz

[1]The market unit may reflect only one arbitrary selected market unit. The marketplace now permits considerable variety.

VOLUME AND WEIGHT OF COMMERCIAL SIZE CONTAINERS

Can Size	Net Weight		Products Package	Approximate Measure	
6 oz	6 oz	170 g	Frozen juices	¾ c	177 ml
8 oz	8 oz	227 g	Concentrates, individual serving juices, vegetables and fruits, tomato paste and sauce	1 c	237 ml
No. 1 Picnic	10½ oz	298 g	Condensed soups, some fruits, vegetables, meat and fish products	1¼ c	296 ml
No.2 Vacuum	12 oz	340 g	Vegetables	1½ c	355 ml
	14½ oz	411 g	Evaporated milk		
	15 oz	425 g	Sweetened condensed milk		
No. 300	15 ½ oz	439 g	Pork and beans, spaghetti, macaroni, chili, date and nut bread, cranberry sauce and blueberries	1¾ c	414 ml
No. 303	15 oz	425 g	Vegetables, fruits	2 c	473 ml
No. 2	20 oz (1 lb 4 oz)	567 g	Juices, vegetables, fruits	2½ c	592 ml
No. 2½	29 oz (1 lb 13oz)	822 g	Fruits, vegetables	3½ c	828 ml
No. 3	46 oz (1 lb 14 fl oz)	1.4 l	Juices whole chicken	5¾ c	1.4 l
No. 10	6 lb 9 oz	3 kg	Institutional or restaurant size for many canned products	3 qt	2.8 l

CHAPTER 13: Food Preservation

DRYING

Some state Cooperative Extension services offer bulletins with instructions for drying foods and for constructing dehydrators. There are a few accurate commercial books available on how to dry foods. Consider the following facts before drying is begun:

- Most fruits and some vegetables, meats, poultry, fish, herbs, nuts, and seeds dry well, but they must be fresh and of high quality to produce a quality product.

- Pretreatment of foods prior to dehydrating is essential. Methods of pre-treating include: ascorbic acid treatment, salt (sodium chloride) solution, or blanching. Blanching can be either in water or steam. Steam blanching is preferred over boiling water for some vegetables because more water-soluble nutrients are retained. Steam blanching requires 50 percent more time than water blanching. Blanching will inactivate enzymes and retard vitamin C loss. Sulfur treatment is not recommended because some individuals are sensitive to it. However, it is useful in preventing discoloration in some fruits, such as apricots. Pretreatment is required for most fruits and vegetables.

- Drying racks may be homemade or commercial, but they should not include such harmful metals as galvanized or cadmium-coated products or copper.

- Drying temperatures must be high enough to prevent foodborne illness but not high enough to cause deterioration of the product. Generally, temperatures between 120°F and 140°F (50–60°C) are used. For best results, use 140°F (60°C).

- Testing for dryness should be done when the food is at room temperature because hot food will respond differently.

- Conditioning the food in a large glass jar for one week after drying will ensure evenness and thoroughness in drying.

- Dried foods are drastically reduced in volume, often one-quarter of the original volume. As a result, they often are consumed in large quantities because they seem small and lightweight, without attention given to their high caloric content and nutrient density.

- Dried foods store well in glass jars in a cool, dry, dark place for maximum shelf life. Containers should be of appropriate size for the amount of food to keep air space to a minimum. Plastic bags sometimes do not protect from insect damage.

- When rehydrating dried foods, any thin liquid that combines well with the food can be used. Examples of liquids are water, milk, fruit juices, bouillon, or ginger ale. For best results with fruit, pour just enough boiling liquid over them to cover. For vegetables, cover and soak in a cold liquid until nearly restored to their original texture. Cover meat with boiling water or broth. Let sit for 30 to 60 minutes, followed by 15 to 20 minutes of simmering before using.

- Regardless of the equipment or techniques used in drying food, vitamin C loss will be significant.

- Microwave ovens are not recommended for drying. The food tends to burn or dry excessively in one spot while being moist in others, and the oven may be damaged.

FOOD FOR DRYING

Most fruits dry well. Those that do not dry well include: avocados and olives because of high fat content; berries (other than strawberries), guavas, and pomegranates because of high seed content; citrus fruits because of juice content and soft pulp; crabapples, quince, and muskmelon because of objectionable flavors when dried. Berries need to be sieved to remove seeds prior to drying to make fruit leather.

- Select firm, ripe fruits. Bruised fruits often can be used in fruit leather after bruises are cut out, but they are not suitable for halves or slices.

- Drying time may vary due to humidity, load, type of food, and efficiency of the dehydrator. The usual range is 3–5 hours for small fruits, 4–7 hours for other fruits except pineapple (8–12 hours).

- Many vegetables are difficult to dry or to rehydrate satisfactorily. Carrots, corn, mushrooms, onions, parsnips, peas, and peppers dry well. These are inexpensive and available fresh year-round, but drying home-grown vegetables is practical and convenient.

- Select absolutely fresh, mature vegetables of high quality. They should be washed well just before drying.

- Drying times will vary from 1–2 hours for herbs, 2–4 hours for other vegetables. The thinner the piece, the shorter the drying time.

- Meat, poultry, or fish should be lean because fat becomes rancid during storage. Meat must be very fresh. Eggs should not be dried in a home dehydrator because quality will be poor.

- Collect herbs for drying as follows: Leaves should be collected just before the plant flowers; flowers should be collected just after the blossoms have opened; seeds should be collected when mature and no longer green.

- Select freshly picked herbs, gathered just after the dew is off. Herbs dry well at room temperature if household dust is not a problem.

- Nuts and seeds are foods naturally preserved by drying. They are usually used in dried form for making desserts and salads or eaten as snacks.

CANNING

Organisms that cause food spoilage — molds, yeast, and bacteria— are always present in the air, water, and soil. Enzymes that may cause undesirable changes in flavor, color, and texture are present in raw fruits and vegetables. When food is canned, it must be processed at a high enough temperature and for a long enough period to destroy any spoilage organisms. This heating process also stops the action of enzymes. The method of canning is determined by the pH, or acidity, of the food.

PRESSURE CANNING

This processing method, utilizing a pressure canner (not a pressure saucepan or steamer), is used for low-acid foods. At sea level, all vegetables (except pickled vegetables), all meat, poultry, and seafood are processed at 10 pounds of pressure with a weighted gauge and 11 pounds with a dial gauge (70 kPa, 240°F or 116°C). Above 1,000 feet in elevation the pressure must be increased to offset the decreasing atmospheric pressure. The higher the elevation, the less atmospheric pressure, hence the lower the boiling point of water. Lower boiling temperatures are less effective in killing bacteria. Increased pressure raises the boiling temperature. *Clostridium botulinum* spores can survive boiling water canner temperatures, but they are killed by the high temperature reached in a pressure canner when processing follows the recommended time and pressure. The pressure canner dial gauge should be tested for accuracy each canning season. County extension offices can provide locations to have the gauge tested. Dial gauges should be replaced if they read inaccurately.

There are two methods of packing vegetables into jars. (See Table 13.1 for specific vegetables.)

Raw Pack — Pack cold, raw vegetables tightly into canning jars or cans and cover with boiling water, wipe the jar rim, and seal with the lid. Place jars in the pressure canner.

Hot Pack — Prepare vegetables by boiling in water a short time (varies with specific vegetable). Loosely fill canning jars with hot vegetable and then add liquid, leaving 1-inch headspace. Wipe the jar rim and adjust lid.

Processing — Follow the manufacturer's directions for the canner being used.

TABLE 13.1
TIMETABLE FOR HOME CANNING VEGETABLES IN PRESSURE CANNER[1,2]

Vegetable	Packing Method	Pint Jar	Quart Jar
Asparagus, 1" (2.5 cm) piece	raw or hot	30 min	40 min
Beans, green, 1" (2.5 cm) piece	raw or hot	20 min	25 min
Beans, lima, fresh	raw or hot	40 min	50 min
Beets, small or sliced	hot	30 min	35 min
Carrots, sliced or diced	raw or hot	25 min	30 min
Corn, cream style	hot	85 min	not recommended
Corn, whole kernel	raw or hot	55 min	85 min
Mushrooms, small, whole, or large, halved or quartered	hot	45 min	not recommended
Okra, cut or whole	hot	25 min	40 min
Peas, green	raw or hot	40 min	40 min
Peppers	hot	35 min	not recommended
Potatoes, small whole	hot	35 min	40 min
Pumpkin, 1" (2.5 cm) cubes	hot	55 min	90 min
Pumpkin, strained	not recommended		
Spinach	hot	70 min	90 min
Squash, winter, 10 (2.5 cm) cubes	hot	55 min	90 min
Squash, winter, strained	not recommended		
Sweet potatoes, cooked	hot	65 min	90 min
Tomato juice	hot	15 min	15 min
Tomatoes, whole or halved	raw or hot	25 min	25 min

[1] At 10 pounds in a weighted gauge canner; 11 pounds in a dial gauge canner (70 kPa, 240°F, or 116°C).

[2] Pressure must be adjusted for altitude by increasing the pressure 1 pound (6.9 kPa) for each 2,000 feet (609 m) above sea level for the dial gauge canner and to 15 pounds (103.4 kPa) for all altitudes above 1,000 feet (304 m) for the weighted-gauge pressure canner.

Here are a few pointers on the use of most pressure canners:

- Preheat two to three inches of water to 180°F (82°C) in the bottom of the canner.

- Set filled jars on rack in pressure canner so that steam can flow around each jar.

- Fasten lid securely so that no steam can escape except through vent (petcock or weighted-gauge opening).

- Watch until steam pours steadily from vent as directed.

- Close petcock or place weighted gauge on vent.

- Let pressure rise to appropriate pounds required for processing. (See Table 13.1.) The moment this pressure is reached, start counting processing time. Keep pressure constant by regulating heat under the canner. Do not lower pressure by opening petcock. Keep drafts from blowing on canner.

- When processing time is up, remove canner from heat immediately. Let canner stand at room temperature until pressure is zero. Never try to rush the cooling. When pressure registers zero, wait two minutes, then slowly open petcock. Unfasten lid and tilt the far side up so that steam escapes away from the body. Remove jars from canner.

- When canning meat, poultry, or seafood, purchase fresh, high quality products and process within 24 hours. When processing homegrown meat or poultry, processing should occur within 24–48 hours after slaughter. The hot pack method of pressure canning is recommended.

- Place large, cut-to-measure pieces of boned, defatted meat in a large shallow pan. Adjust enough water to keep meat from sticking. Cover and cook slowly on top of the range or in a 350°F (180°C) oven until the meat is medium done or it reaches an internal temperature of 155°F (68°C), turning it occasionally so it precooks evenly.

- Pack hot meat loosely in a jar, leaving one inch (2.5 cm) headspace. Add 1 teaspoon (5 ml) salt per quart (1 l) if desired. Add boiling meat juice (extended with boiling water if necessary), leaving one inch (2.5 cm) of headspace. Wipe jar rims thoroughly; adjust lids according to manufacturer's instructions.

- Pressure-process at 90 minutes at 10 pounds pressure with a weighted gauge; 11 pounds with a dial gauge (70 kPa, 240°F, or 116°C). Be sure to adjust for altitude.

BOILING WATER CANNER METHOD

This processing method is used for all acid foods: fruits, tomatoes with added acid, jams, jellies, and pickled vegetables. The canner must be at least four inches (10cm) higher than the tops of the jars. It needs a lid and wire rack. A pressure canner may be used, with the petcock left wide open to prevent pressure buildup. See Table 13.2 for correct processing time. As is also true for pressure canning, never use a jar unless it is a canning jar.

Pack food either raw or hot:

Raw Pack — Put raw fruits into container and cover with boiling hot syrup, juice, or water. Press tomatoes down in the containers so they are covered with their own juice. (See directions below for hot pack for acidifying tomatoes.)

Hot Pack — Heat fruits in syrup, water, or steam, or in extracted juice before packing. Juicy fruits and tomatoes may be preheated without added liquid and packed in the juice of cooked fruit. To acidify tomatoes, add two tablespoons (30 ml) of bottled lemon juice or ½ teaspoon (3 ml) of citric acid per quart (l) of tomatoes.

Sugar syrup concentrations used in canning fruits are as follows:

- Fill jars, leaving ½ inch (1.2 cm) headspace. Put on cap, screw band firmly. Put filled and capped glass jars into half-filled water bath canner of preheated water, 140°F (60°C) for raw pack and 180°F (82°C) for hot-packed foods.

- Add boiling water, if needed, to bring water an inch or two (2.5 – 5 cm) over tops of jars. Do not pour boiling water directly on glass jars. Put lid on canner.

- When water in canner comes to a rolling boil, start to count processing time. (See Table 13.2.) Boil gently and steadily for the time recommended for the food being canned. Add boiling water during processing, if needed, to keep jars covered. Immediately remove jars from the canner when processing time is complete.

- Cool overnight before testing for seal and removing screws bands. Wash jars, dry, label, and store without bands.

See Table 13.3 for estimation of yield and jars needed for canning fruits and vegetables.

Sugar Type	Sugar %	Water		Sugar		Yield	
				c	ml	c	l
Very light	10	6½	1.6	¾	175	6¾	1.6
Light	20	5¾	1.4	1½	375	6½	1.5
Medium	30	5¼	1.3	2¼	550	6	1.4
Heavy	40	5	1.2	3¼	800	6½	1.5
Very heavy	50	4¼	1.0	4¼	1050	6½	1.5

TABLE 13.2
BOILING WATER CANNER PROCESSING

Food Item	Style of Pack	Jar Size	Time in Minutes			
			0-1000 (0-304 m)	1001-3000 (303-913 m)	3001-6000 (914-1826 m)	Above 6000 (1826 m +)
Apple slices	hot	pt	20	25	30	35
		qt	20	25	30	35
Applesauce	hot	pt	15	20	20	25
		qt	20	25	30	35
Apricots, peaches, nectarines	hot	pt	20	25	30	35
		qt	25	30	35	40
	raw	pt	25	30	35	40
		qt	30	35	40	45

BOILING WATER CANNER PROCESSING (CONTINUED)

Food Item	Style of Pack	Jar Size	Time in Minutes			
			0-1000 (0-304 m)	1001-3000 (303-913 m)	3001-6000 (914-1826 m)	Above 6000 (1826 m +)
Berries	hot	pt	15	20	20	25
		qt	15	20	20	25
	raw	pt	15	20	20	25
		qt	20	25	30	35
Cherries	hot	pt	15	20	20	25
		qt	20	25	30	35
	raw	pt	25	30	35	40
		qt	25	30	35	40
Fruit puree except figs and tomatoes	hot	pt	15	20	20	25
		qt	15	20	20	25
Grapefruit, orange sections	raw	pt	10	15	15	20
		qt	10	15	15	20
Pears	hot	pt	20	25	30	35
		qt	25	30	35	40
Plums	hot/ raw	pt	20	25	30	35
		qt	25	30	35	40
Rhubarb	hot	pt	15	20	20	25
		qt	15	20	20	25
Tomato juice	hot	pt	35	40	45	50
		qt	45	50	55	60
Tomato whole/halved / Tomato water pack	hot/ raw	pt	40	45	50	55
		qt	45	50	55	60
Tomato whole/halved / Tomato juice pack	hot/ raw	pt	85	90	95	100
		qt	85	90	95	100
Tomato no added liquid	raw	pt	85	90	95	100
		qt	85	90	95	100
Jams and jellies	hot	½ pt pt	5	10	10	15

BOILING WATER CANNER PROCESSING (CONTINUED)

Food Item	Style of Pack	Jar Size	Time in Minutes			
			0-1000 (0-304 m)	1001-3000 (303-913 m)	3001-6000 (914-1826 m)	Above 6000 (1826 m +)
Spreads	hot	½ pt	15	20	20	25
		pt	20	30	30	35
Dill pickles	raw	pt	10	15	15	20
		qt	15	20	20	25
Bread & butter pickles	hot	pt	10	15	15	20
		qt	10	15	15	20
14-day sweet pickles	raw	pt	5	10	10	15
		qt	10	15	15	20
Sauerkraut	hot	pt	10	15	15	20
		qt	15	20	20	25
	raw	pt	20	25	30	35
		qt	25	30	35	40

PICKLES AND RELISHES

For all pickle and relish products, processing in the boiling water canner is recommended. (See Table 13.2 for recommended times.) **DO NOT USE OPEN KETTLE CANNING.**

- Use vinegar with five to six percent acidity. Canning and pickling salt should be used for all brines.

- Processing times for relishes depend on the combination of vegetables. Obtain a USDA recipe to ensure safety.

- For brined or fermented pickles, use a USDA recipe and a fermenting time of two to four weeks.

- For fresh pack pickles, cure them in brine for several hours or overnight.

- For relishes prepared from fruits and vegetables, chop, season, and then cook. Hot pack.

- For fruit pickles, prepare them from whole fruits and simmer in a spicy, sweet-sour syrup. Hot pack.

CAUTION: Developing one's own recipes and using combinations of foods are not recommended in home canning. Instead, freeze the product. Only recipes based on USDA recommendations should be used. Changing ingredients can result in different density and acidity, resulting in an under-processed and unsafe food.

JELLIES AND JAMS

Jelly, jam, conserve, marmalade, and preserves are all fruit products that add zest to meals. These methods provide a way to use inferior fruit (the largest or smallest fruits and berries and those that are irregularly shaped) that are not suitable for canning or freezing. Basically, these products are similar; all of them are preserved by means of sugar and usually gelled to some extent. Pectin, sugar, and acid levels of fruit vary, making it impossible to develop formulas that will always give the same results. In products made with pectin, use ¼ to ½ cup (50 to 125 ml) more fruit or juice to make a softer product. Use ¼ to ½ cup (50 to 125 ml) less fruit or juice to make a firmer product. In products made without added pectin, a shorter cooking time gives a softer product. Lengthen the cooking time for a firmer product.

Jelly is made from fruit juice; the product is clear and firm enough to hold its shape when turned out of the container.

Jam is made from crushed or ground fruit. It tends to hold its shape but generally is less firm than jelly. Freezer jam is made with added pectin and is not processed. The taste and color are more like fresh fruit.

Conserves are jams made from a mixture of fruits, usually including citrus fruits; often raisins and nuts are added.

Marmalade is a tender jelly with small pieces of fruit distributed evenly throughout. Marmalade commonly contains citrus fruit.

Preserves are whole fruits or large pieces of fruit in a thick syrup, often slightly gelled.

Fruit butter is a smooth, less sweet preserve made from fruit pulp run through a sieve and cooked slowly.

Some fruits have enough natural pectin to make high-quality products. These fruits are citrus, some apples, grapes, blackberries, boysenberries, cranberries, and some plums. Other fruits require added pectin for making jellies that are firm enough to hold their shape. These fruits are peaches, pears, apricots, elderberries, strawberries, and raspberries. All fruits have less pectin when they are fully ripe than when they are underripe.

Commercial fruit pectins made from apples or citrus fruits are on the market in both liquid and powdered form. Either form is satisfactory when used in a recipe developed especially for that form. Commercial pectins can lose their gelling capabilities if stored too long or cooked too long when preparing the product. Unused pectin should be stored in a cool dry place.

The advantages of using pectin are that fully ripe fruit can be used, cooking time is short, and the yield is greater.

The acid content varies in different fruits and is higher in underripe fruits. With fruits low in acid, lemon juice or citric acid commonly is added to make gelled products. Commercial fruit pectins contain some acid. Lemon juice is usually added to increase acid content of fruit. If desired, ⅛ teaspoon (0.6 ml) of citric acid can be substituted for each tablespoon (15 ml) of lemon juice.

When using cane or beet sugar, the ratio of sugar to fruit is ¾/4:1 for most fruits. It is best to add sugar before cooking. Sugar helps in gel formation, serves as a preserving agent, and contributes to the flavor. It also has a firming effect on fruit, a property that is useful in the making of preserves. To use corn syrup or honey in jelly making, use a tested recipe to ensure success.

Gelling tests for making jelly without pectin are:

Spoon or sheet test: dip a cool metal spoon in boiling jelly, then carry it out of the steam and pour from the spoon. Jelly is done when syrup forms two drops that flow together and sheet off the edge of the spoon.

Freezer test: remove jelly from heat. Pour a small amount of boiling jelly on a cold plate and place in freezer. When it is cooled, see if it is gelled.

To make jelly with pectin using the short-boil method, mix powdered pectin with unheated fruit juice, bring mixture to a boil, add sugar, and boil for one minute at a full boil. If using liquid pectin, add it to the boiling juice and sugar mixture and boil for one minute at a full rolling boil. Follow directions for the specific product.

Filling and sealing containers when jelly is done:

For jelly, fill to ¼ inch (0.6 cm) from top and seal. Process according to instructions in Table 13.2.

For sweet spreads, let stand 5 minutes, stirring occasionally to keep fruit from floating. Place in jars and seal. Then process in boiling water canner according to instructions in Table 13.2.

Reduced-sugar fruit spreads are made with several different gelling or thickening agents, each of which gives somewhat different characteristics to the product. Reduced or no sugar may be used. Sweet fruits, apple juice, and/or a liquid low-calorie or non-caloric sweetener may be added for flavor. Preservation is dependent on the boiling water canner processing, refrigerator storage, or frozen storage. Directions given for the commercial thickening ingredient being used should be followed. If unflavored gelatin powder is used as the gelling agent, the products must be refrigerated and used within four weeks.

TABLE 13.3
ESTIMATION OF YIELD AND JARS NEEDED FOR CANNING FRUITS AND VEGETABLES

Raw Produce	Measures	Approximate Number	Approximate Pounds
		Quart (950 ml) Jars Needed	Needed for 1 Quart Jar
Fruits			
Apples	1 bu. (48 lb)	16–20	2½ to 3
Applesauce	1 bu. (48 lb)	15–18	2½ to 3½
Apricots	1 lug (22 lb)	7–11	2 to 2½
Berries	24-quart crate	12–18	1½ to 3
Cherries	1 bu. (56 lb)	22–33 (unpitted)	2 to 2½
	1 lug (22 lb)	9–11	2 to 2½
Peaches	1 bu. (48 lb)	18–24	2 to 3
	1 lug (22 lb)	8–12	2 to 3
Pears	1 bu. (50 lb)	20–25	2 to 3
	1 box (35 lb)	14–17	2 to 3
Plums	1 bu. (56 lb)	24–30	1½ to 2½
	1 lug (24 lb)	12	1½ to 2½
Tomatoes	1 bu. (53 lb)	15–20	2½ to 3½
	1 lug (30 lb)	10	2½ to 3½
Tomatoes for juice	1 bu. (53 lb)	12–16	3 to 3½

ESTIMATION OF YIELD AND JARS NEEDED FOR CANNING
FRUITS AND VEGETABLES (CONTINUED)

Raw Produce	Measures	Approximate Number Quart (950 ml) Jars Needed	Approximate Pounds Needed for 1 Quart Jar
Vegetables			
Beans, lima (in pods)	1 bu. (32 lb)	6 – 10	3 to 5
Beans, green or wax	1 bu. (30 lb)	12 – 20	1½ to 2½
Beets (without tops)	1 bu. (52 lb)	15 – 24	2 to 3½
Carrots (without tops)	1 bu. (50 lb)	16 – 25	2 to 3
Corn, sweet (in husks)	1 bu. (35 lb)	6 – 10 (whole kernel)	3 to 6
Okra	1 bu. (26 lb)	16 – 18	1½
Peas (in pods)	1 bu. (30 lb)	5 – 10	3 to 6
Spinach and other greens	1 bu. (18 lb)	3 – 8	2 to 6
Squash, summer	1 bu. (40 lb)	10 – 20	2 to 4
Sweet potatoes	1 bu. (50 lb)	18–25	2 to 3

NOTE: The actual number of jars needed in canning depends on the size and condition of the produce and the manner of preparing and packing into jars. The standard weight of a bushel, lug, or box is not the same in all states.

FREEZING

Freezing preserves many foods with little change in flavor, color, texture, and nutritional value. Freezing, one of the simplest methods of home food preservation, does not sterilize the product; it simply retards the growth of harmful bacteria and molds. Therefore, good sanitation procedures are necessary for freezing. The wrapping or container for the food that is being frozen is very important. Boxes, jars, and bags especially made for freezing are available. A freezer container or wrap should:

- Be impermeable to oxygen
- Be odorless
- Possess high wet strength
- Be grease-proof
- Be non-adherent to the frozen product
- Be puncture resistant
- Be easy to mark
- Not crack at low temperature

Plastic freezer containers or other sealed rigid containers are preferred for liquid packs. Canning jars designed for freezing and used with home canning lids are excellent for freezing liquids. Jars are easily resealed after removing a portion of their contents. Allow enough headspace for expansion of liquid during freezing to prevent breakage. Be sure to follow manufacturer's directions.

Flexible bags or wrappings of moisture/vapor-resistant polyethylene, cellophane, nylon, or plastic are suitable for dry-pack vegetables, fruits, meats, poultry, and fish. Bags also may be used for liquid packs, but breakage and leakage should be expected.

Laminated freezer papers made of various combinations of paper, foil, or plastic are suitable for dry-pack meats, fish, and poultry. Metal foils are easily torn or punctured.

BASIC STEPS IN FREEZING

- Use only quality fresh products.

- Work under very sanitary conditions.

- Organize everything that is needed to save time and energy.

- Use appropriate packing materials.

- Follow directions for the product being frozen: blanch or scald vegetables; blanch 1 minute longer at 5000 feet (1524 m) and above; cool quickly, use ascorbic acid for light –colored fruits to prevent discoloration, use appropriate pack for fruits, keep meats cold while preparing for freezing.

- Package, removing all air.

- Label with date and name of product.

- Promptly place in freezer in single layers.

- Maintain 0°F (–18°C) in freezer.

- Keep an inventory.

- Use all products within recommended storage period for best quality.

HOW TO PACK FRUITS

Fruits should be slightly riper than they are for canning. Fruits can be packed in syrup or dry sugar. The intended use of the fruit will determine the type of pack used. Forty percent syrup is recommended for most fruits. (See Table 13.4 for quantities needed.)

- Syrup pack: dissolve sugar in water until solution is clear. Use just enough cool syrup to cover the fruit in the container. Allow ½ inch (1.2 cm) headspace.

- Sugar pack: works well for soft fruits such as strawberries. Add sugar to clean prepared fruits. Let stand 10 to 15 minutes. Stir to coat each piece. Pack fruit tightly in storage containers.

- Dry pack: pack fruit in containers without sugar or syrup. No headspace is necessary.

- Individual quick frozen (IQF): this pack is good for small whole fruit. The fruit is frozen individually without sugar on a shallow metal tray or cookie sheet and then packed in a container for storage.

- Ascorbic acid should be used with fruits that tend to darken quickly (peaches, apricots, figs, sweet cherries, pears, and apples). Follow manufacturer's directions as to method and amount.

Freezing fruit allows jelly- and jam-making anytime of the year.

Refer to Table 13.4 for information on percent recovery.

Type of Syrup %	Sugar		Water		Amount of Syrup	
	c	l	c	l	c	l
30	2	0.5	4	1	5	1.2
40	3	0.8	4	1	5½	1.4
50	4¾	1.2	4	1	6½	1.6
60	7	1.8	4	1	7¾	1.9

TABLE 13.4

WEIGHT CONVERSIONS: FARM TO PROCESSED FROZEN FRUITS

Frozen Fruits	% Recovery	Frozen Weight from Farm Weight[1]
Apples	60	0.60
Apricots	78	0.91
Berries		
Blackberries	95	0.95
Blueberries	97	0.97
Boysenberries	88	0.88
Gooseberries	97	0.97
Loganberries	88	0.88
Raspberries	95	0.95
Strawberries	93	1.12
Cherries		
sour	75	0.90
sweet	85	0.85
Grapes	85	0.85
Peaches	67	0.80
Pineapples	50	0.625

[1] Frozen weight is weight of frozen fruits plus sugar content. Fruit to sugar ratio is used in this computation: apricots 6 to 1; strawberries, sour cherries, peaches, 5 to 1; pineapples, 4 to 1; other fruits, 0.

VEGETABLES

Speed from garden to freezer is the important factor in vegetable freezing. Blanching destroys enzymes that will cause deterioration of quality and vitamin C loss during storage. Blanching also cleanses the surface of microorganisms and softens the product, which makes it easier to package. Vegetables are lowered into boiling water or in steam for a specific amount of time and then quickly cooled before packing to freeze. (See Table 13.5 for blanching times.)

Vegetables for freezing can be packed in two ways.

Dry Pack — After vegetables have been blanched, cooled, and drained, place them in meal-size, airtight, moisture-proof containers. After packaging, remove all air possible from the container before it is sealed. Allow headspace for expansion of the vegetables during freezing.

Individual Quick Frozen (IQF) — After vegetable pieces have been blanched, cooled, and drained, spread them in a single layer on shallow trays or pans. Place trays in the freezer for four to six hours, then quickly package frozen pieces in a suitable resealable container. Unblanched diced onions and peppers may be IQF packed.

TABLE 13.5
TIMETABLE FOR BLANCHING VEGETABLES PRIOR TO FREEZING

Vegetable	Minutes Heated in Boiling Water[1,2]	Vegetable	Minutes Heated in Boiling Water[1,2]
Asparagus		**Broccoli**	
small stalks	1½	florets 1½ inches (3.8 cm) in diameter	3
medium stalks	2	large	4
large stalks	3	**Brussels sprouts**	
Beans, lima		small heads	3
small beans or pods	1	medium	4
medium beans or pods	2	large	5
large beans or pods	3	**Cabbage**	
Beans, wax or green	3	coarse shreds or thin wedges	1½
Beets		wedges	3
small	25 to 30		
medium	45 to 50		

TIMETABLE FOR BLANCHING VEGETABLES PRIOR TO FREEZING (CONTINUED)

Vegetable	Minutes Heated in Boiling Water[1,2]
Carrots	
whole small	5
diced, sliced, strips	3
Cauliflower	
medium	3
large	4
Corn, sweet	
small ears — 1¼ inches (3 cm) or less in diameter	5
medium ears — 1¼ to 1½ inches (3–3.8 cm) in diameter	6
large ears — 1½ to 2 inches (3–5 cm) in diameter	8
extra large ears—over 2 inches (5 cm) in diameter	10
whole kernel	5 to 6
Greens, all types	2
Kohlrabi	
½ inch (1.2 cm) cubes	2
whole, small to medium	3
Okra	
small pods	3
large pods	5

Vegetable	Minutes Heated in Boiling Water[1,2]
Parsnips, ½ inch (1.2 cm) cubes or slices	5
Peas	
black-eyed	
small	1
large	2
green	2
Pumpkin	until soft
Rutabagas, ½ inch (1.2 cm) cubes	3
Squash	
summer, 1½ inch (1.2 cm) slices	3
winter	until soft
Sweet potatoes	until soft
Tomatoes	
whole	until soft
juice, simmer tomatoes	5
Turnips, ½ inch (1.2 cm) cubes	3

[1]For each pound of prepared vegetable, use at least 1 gallon of boiling water. After heating for the specified time, cool promptly in cold water and drain.

[2]Adjust time for altitude so under-blanching does not occur.

MEAT

Freezing is the best method of meat storage. Starting with a wholesome, high-quality product will ensure the best results. All meat should be wrapped in moisture-vapor-proof material that is impermeable to oxygen.

THAWING

With the exception of spinach and corn-on-the-cob, vegetables may be taken directly from the freezer, unpacked, and steamed or boiled. Spinach and corn-on-the-cob are better if first thawed in a microwave oven or in the refrigerator for four hours.

Meats, fish, shellfish, and vegetables should not be thawed at room temperature. Many bacteria on fresh food will still be present when food is thawed. The nutrients in the drip that forms upon thawing support rapid bacterial growth. Bacteria capable of causing illness are common on vegetables, meats, poultry, and seafood. Improper thawing of these products may lead to illness. Thawing sealed packages of foods rapidly in cold water is an acceptable practice, but the cold water should be changed every 5 to 10 minutes. Proper thawing will help ensure safe food. Leftover frozen foods should be held below 40°F or above 140°F (4°–60°C) to avoid possible foodborne illnesses.

FOODS NOT SUITABLE FOR FREEZING

Some foods not suitable for freezing are raw cabbage, cake batters, raw celery, cream pie fillings, custards, cooked egg whites, lettuce, mayonnaise, potato salad, salad dressing, fresh tomatoes, and watermelon.

IF FREEZER STOPS

If the power fails or the freezer stops operating normally, try to determine how long it will be before the freezer will be back in operation.

A fully-loaded freezer usually will stay cold enough to keep foods frozen for two days if the cabinet is not opened. In a cabinet with less than half a load, food may not stay frozen more than one day. Some partially thawed foods can be refrozen. Generally, refreezing should not pose a health hazard if the food has not reached 40°F (4°C). If thawed food still contains a few ice crystals, it is safe to refreeze. Quality loss occurs with thawing and refreezing. However, it is least evident in red meats and most evident in fish and seafood.

Meat, poultry and vegetables — Refreeze if the temperature is 40°F (4°C) or below and if the color and odor are good. Discard packages that show signs of spoilage, such as off-colors or bad odors.

Fruits — Refreeze if they smell and taste good. Thawed fruits also may be used in cooking or making jellies, jams, and preserves.

Cooked foods — Refreeze if ice crystals are still present or the freezer is 40°F (4°C) or below. If the condition is poor or questionable, throw it out.

If normal operation cannot be resumed before the food will start to thaw, use dry ice. If dry ice is placed in the freezer soon after the power is off, 25 pounds (11 kg) should keep the temperature below freezing for two to three days in a 10-cubic-foot (0.3 m3) cabinet with half a load, and three to four days in a loaded cabinet. Place the dry ice on cardboard or small boards on top of packages and do not open cabinet again except to put in more dry ice or to remove it when normal operation is resumed.

Another suggestion is to move the food to a locker plant, using insulated boxes or thick layers of paper to prevent thawing while in transit. The locker plant can refreeze the packaged food more quickly, resulting in better quality.

Index